The Influence of the Pharmaceutical Industry on Medicine, as Exemplified by Proton Pump Inhibitors

The Influence of the Pharmaceutical Industry on Medicine, as Exemplified by Proton Pump Inhibitors

By

Helge L. Waldum

Cambridge Scholars Publishing

The Influence of the Pharmaceutical Industry on Medicine, as Exemplified by Proton Pump Inhibitors

By Helge L. Waldum

This book first published 2020

Cambridge Scholars Publishing

Lady Stephenson Library, Newcastle upon Tyne, NE6 2PA, UK

British Library Cataloguing in Publication Data
A catalogue record for this book is available from the British Library

ISBN (10): 1-5275-5882-7
ISBN (13): 978-1-5275-5882-3

Contents

ACKNOWLEDGEMENTS

I am grateful to my parents and my whole family for raising me to become independent and self-confident. I appreciate the money given to me by the Cancer Foundation at St. Olavs Hospital and I wish to particularly thank Ove Mjølnerød who was its chairman for many years. For many years, this foundation was the sole founder of my research. I am also indebted to my 20 PhD candidates, who contributed to a solid foundation for the research. Among them, I would particularly like to mention my first PhD candidate, Per Martin Kleveland, who, together with the pediatric surgeon Stein Haugen, contributed to the development of the isolated rat stomach model. I am also grateful to the technicians working within the unit. Furthermore, I am grateful to Eiliv Brenna, who nominated me to become a Knight of St. Olav's Order, and to Irvin Modlin and Kristian Bjøro for writing the required recommendations.

During my career, I spent 8 years in the far north, Tromsø, where Professor Per Burhol immediately guided me into the field of gastroenterology because, on my very first day, he told me that I should start research on gastrin (January 2, 1974). Since then, I have devoted all of my energy to this field, and I am very grateful because, as I see it, the stomach and gastrin are ideal research areas which may make important contributions to physiology and diseases, particularly with regard to tumorigenesis. Since 1981, I have worked at the University Hospital in Trondheim where Professor Hermod Petersen helped me to establish my research; he also provided excellent clinical facilities. I also spent a year in Paris at the Hôpital Bichat, which was headed by Professor Serge Bonfils, who inspired me to focus on basic science and devote my research to trophic regulation, which later led to my interest in tumorigenesis. I would also like to express my gratitude to the head of my institute, Torstein Baade Rø, for letting me continue as a professor even though I was over 72 years old.

I am grateful to my first wife Christin for teaching me how to behave. Finally, I would like to express my gratitude to my wife, Wilma, for her support, patience and, particularly, her technical help.

My 20 PhD Candidates

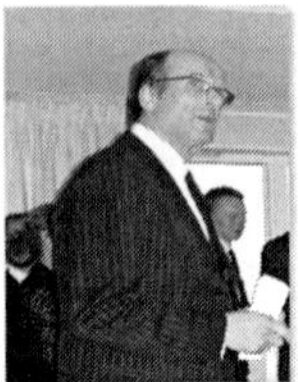

Per Martin Kleveland

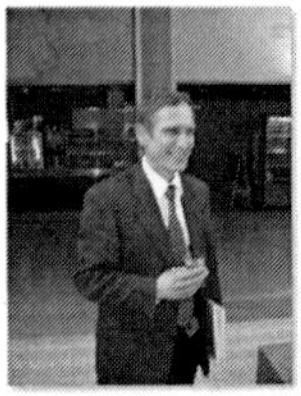

Arne Sandvik

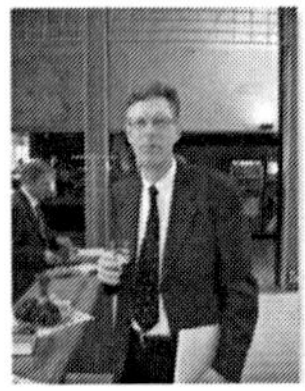

Eiliv Brenna

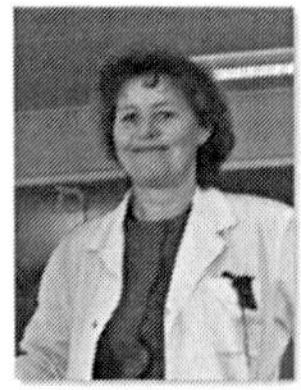

Unni Syversen

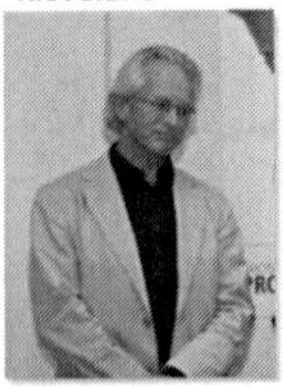

Anders Angelsen

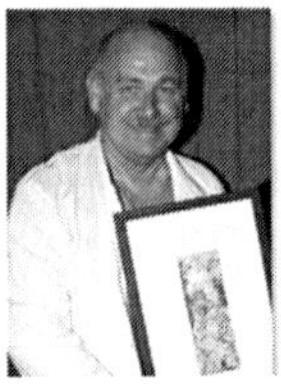

Ronald Mårvik

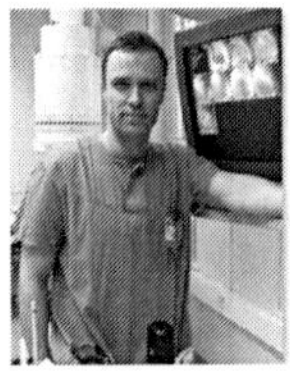

Gunnar Qvigstad

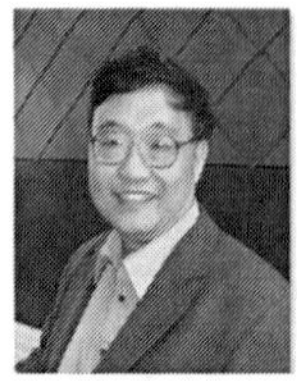

Guanglin Cui

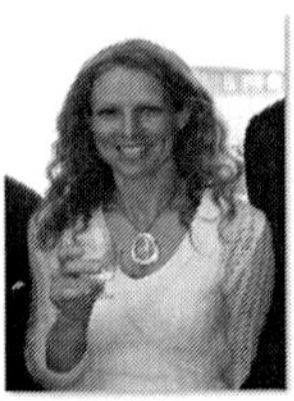

Ingunn Bakke

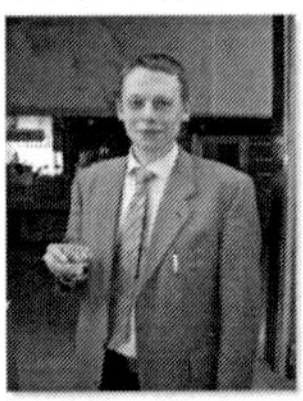

Tom Chr. Martinsen

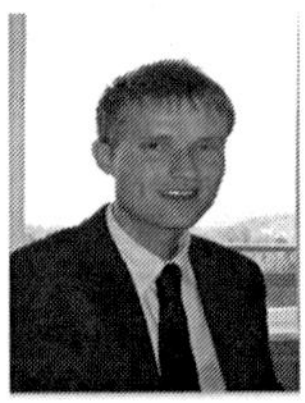

Reidar Fossmark

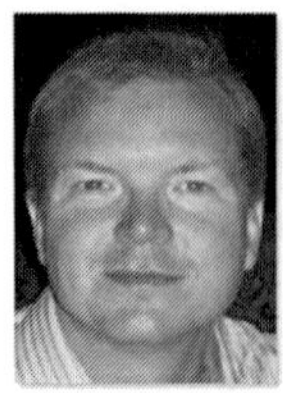

Björn Gustafsson

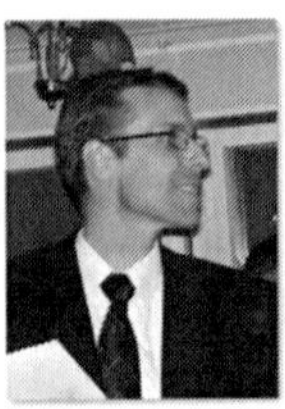

Sveinung Sørhaug

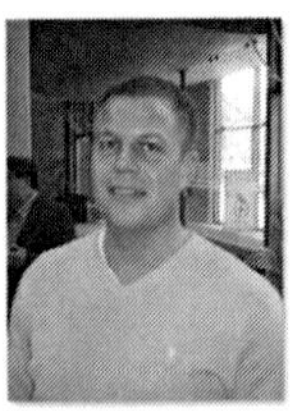

Øyvind Hauso

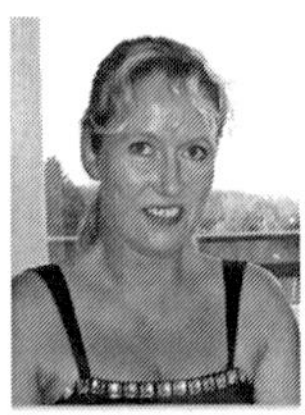

Karin E. Bakkelund

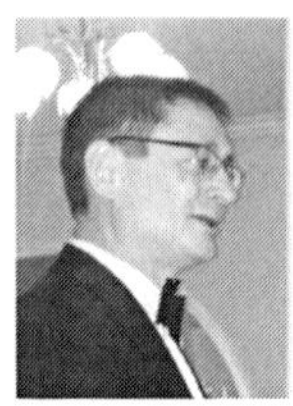

Constantin S. Jianu

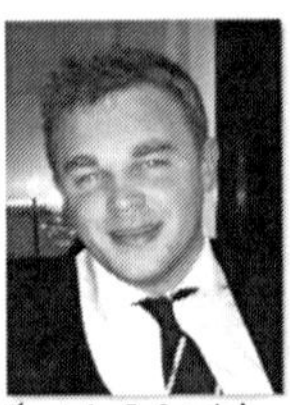

Øystein F. Sørdal

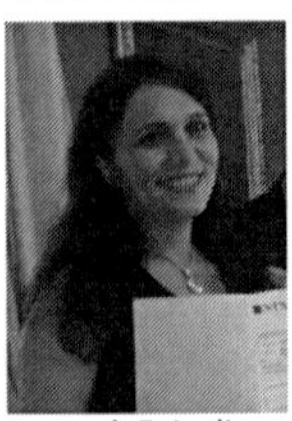

Fatemeh Zeinali

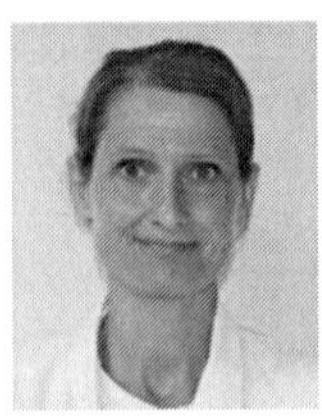

Liv Sagatun

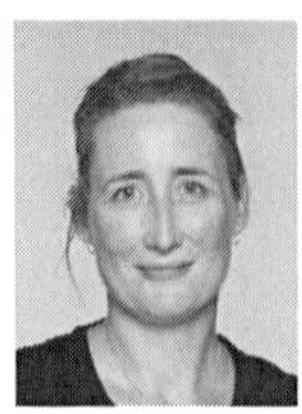

Patricia Mjønes

PREFACE

During my long clinical and scientific career, I have met with a lot of obstruction, which has not appeared to be scientifically based. During my younger years, I was surprised to see how doctors and scientists took the side of the pharmaceutical industry, but over time I have learnt that this is, unfortunately, the usual way.

I have also realized that the pharmaceutical industry is not interested in long-term side effects. This attitude has gained traction by relying solely on "evidence-based medicine", which does not say anything about long-term side effects. Using statements such as "a man is not a rat" suppresses the importance of animal toxicology studies, despite the fact that long-term animal studies are the only way to detect late occurring side effects before they occur in patients.

My experience is based on gastric physiology and gastroenterology, but I feel certain that similar experiences may be gained in other parts of medicine. I hope that this short book will show that the pharmaceutical industry suppresses any discussion on long-term side effects, and that most doctors and scientists within the area are willing to adjust their work to please industrial interests.

Helgc L. Waldum
Professor of Medicine,
Norwegian University of Science and Technology,
Trondheim, Norway

CHAPTER 1

BACKGROUND

Abstract

My family background, education, and career are described. I also mention the people who have guided me and who I have collaborated with in the field of gastric physiology and pathology. Professor Per G. Burhol in Tromsø guided me into clinical gastroenterology and research. On my first day at work at Tromsø Hospital, he told me that I should study gastrin and I have continued to pursue this area for 45 years. I am very happy with my decision to do so because the stomach is an ideal organ to study because the gastric juice is useful for both animal and human biological studies. Moreover, due to the fact that gastric juice primarily kills microorganisms, apart from Helicobacter pylori, the results are not influenced by infections. Later, I was inspired by Professor Hermod Petersen in Trondheim, and then, in Paris, Professor Serge Bonfils made me consider how gastrin's trophic effects could pave my way into tumor research. Professor Jens Rehfeld helped me establish radioimmunoassays for gastrointestinal hormones, and Professor Rolf Håkanson assisted me in the creation of new methods for studying the regulation of gastric acid secretion. Finally, Sir James Black was a friend and an inspiration. My friendship with him allowed me early access to the gastrin antagonist, netazepide. Black believed that this compound could be his third most important drug following the first β-blocker and the first histamine-2 blocker.

Keywords: animal studies; gastric acid; gastric physiology; gastric pathology; gastrin; inhibitors of gastric acid secretion; isolated rat stomach; long-term side effects; pharmaceutical companies.

I was born in rural Norway one year after the Second World War ended. My father was a worker and my mother, the daughter of a farmer, was a housewife. I have a brother who is six years older than me, who was born at the start of the war in Norway. I was the result of peace and optimism. My parents built a new house on my mother's father's land. We moved into the new house shortly before I was born. I grew up close to my grandparents and their three sons and daughter, who were all unmarried at that time. Moreover, my grandfather's brother and his wife lived at the same farm. They had no children. The small farm where my father grew up was run by my father's brother and sister. I was the only young child among a lot of relatives who adored me.

My grandfather and his brother taught me that a man should be tough and strong and do heavy manual work. Office work was not regarded as real work for a man. At the same time, my parents and relatives were interested in politics, and in the late evenings I remember sitting on my father's lap listening to parliamentary debates on the radio. I was cared for by all my relatives as I was the youngest child. For instance, my grandfather's childless brother would not wake me up if I fell asleep on his lap. He would wait until I woke up before he started his work on the farm. This meant that I had a lot of self-confidence during my early childhood. However, I was not spoiled, and I knew that I needed to excel to reach my goals. Fortunately, I was good at both sport and schoolwork. My elder brother let me play sport with him and his friends. I had a talent for soccer and cross-country skiing, which are the most important sports in Norway. Now I joke that if I was still young then I would play soccer instead of being a doctor. Mathematics was my favorite subject at school, along with history and related subjects. My interests were helped by the discussions I was having at home.

At school, I was always among the best pupils at each level. I moved to the small town of Steinkjer at sixteen years old. Moving away from home was perhaps good for my professional career, but harmful for my sporting activities. After three years, I passed my exams, but I did not get top marks in my favorite subjects, mathematics and physics, despite having the correct answers. However, I received top marks in English, which was never one of my best subjects. I received the marks required to study medicine at the University of Oslo. During my six years in Oslo, I met my first wife and had my first child. Every time I moved to another school, I thought that I would meet students who were brighter than me. However, I continued to excel and when I was in Oslo passed a degree with such good marks that it was reported to the King. This was based on hard work and the fact that I never left anything without understanding it. If there was something I did not understand, I would attempt to make my own hypothesis. I enjoyed working as a young doctor at the hospital in Molde and as general practitioner in the community. However, I wanted to work in a hospital, preferably performing a combination of clinical work and research.

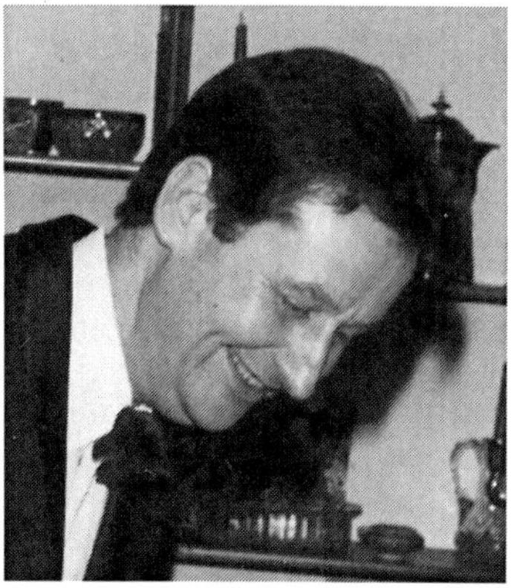

Professor Per G. Burhol
(Photo: private)

After a short stay in Oslo, I moved to Tromsø where a new university had just been established, which had plenty of money but needed devoted people. Some months before my arrival in Tromsø, Professor Per G. Burhol had become the head of gastroenterology (Burhol et al. 1982) He had seen my good marks at the University of Oslo and immediately offered me a position in gastroenterology, which combined clinical work and research. He said that I should start researching gastrin, and so I went to Copenhagen to learn about gastrin radioimmunoassay from Professor Jens F. Rehfeld (Rehfeld 1973).

This went well and after six years I was a specialist in internal medicine with a subspecialty in gastroenterology and had made research sufficient to become a professor. I then became the Head of the Department during my last year in Tromsø. Here, I learned the value of frank discussions and openness, particularly from Professor Arne Nordøy (von Houwelingen et al. 1987).

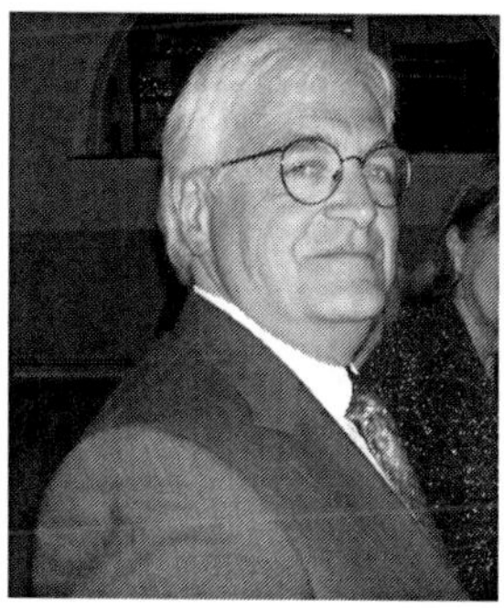

Professor Jens F. Rehfeld
(Photo: private)

Coming from a farming family, I felt that the soil in Tromsø was too barren, and so I moved Trondheim in the middle of Norway, which is close to the valley where I grew up. Since then, I have lived in Trondheim, apart from one sabbatical year in Paris in 1987–88. I chose France because I had been Francophile since my childhood when I listened to the dramatic events that took place during the fifties on the radio. I enjoyed the warm and long summer in Paris but felt that the winter was a little dull compared with the snow in Norway.

In Paris, I worked at Hôpital Bichat, which was led by the "King" of French gastroenterology, Professor Serge Bonfils (Bonfils, Mignon, and Accary 1975). While I was there, I fulfilled a course in basic science with a focus on the gastrointestinal tract. It included two written and two oral examinations and, once you had passed these tests, you could start your thesis. This course not only benefitted me scientifically, but it also enabled me to learn the language. I also realized during a discussion in one of the oral examinations that I had to study not only the physiological role of gastrin with respect to gastric acid secretion, but also gastrin's role in the regulation of the growth and development of tumors. These subjects became my main interests, and the quarrel I had with Bonfils during my examination was later a great help.

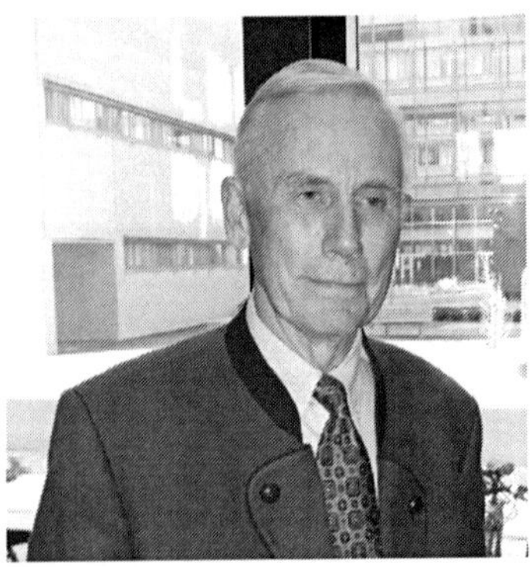

Professor Hermod Petersen
(Photo: private)

When I came from Tromsø to Trondheim, I immediately received support from Professor Hermod Petersen (Petersen 1969), who made me a senior consultant and then later a professor. I was given my professorship by the King, which made me an officer of the Crown. However, not long after this, professors lost that title. Together with my first candidate, Professor Per M. Kleveland; an eminent pediatric surgeon, Stein Haugen; and Arne Sandvik we established the completely isolated rat stomach model, and made it produce acid (Kleveland et al. 1986). This breakthrough in gastric physiology was partly due to a membrane oxygenator, which was produced by the Department of Technology at our university. Soon afterwards, we came across the first reliable method to determine histamine concentrations. We applied this method on blood from the stomach and, in doing so, we were able to study the effects of substances added to the arterial side on gastric acid secretion, as well as the release of signal substances to the blood.

Our manuscripts based upon these new methods were turned down, and even met with hostility, which of course was a great disappointment. However, I have come to learn that the most popular manuscripts are the ones that support the view of certain influential "gurus" within the field. New findings, even if they are supported experimentally, tend to be discarded. It has been especially problematic to have studies accepted within pathology that cast doubt upon current tumor classifications. I went into pathology after my stay in France, as I was interested in the tumors that occur in rodents after the long-term inhibition of gastric acid secretion.

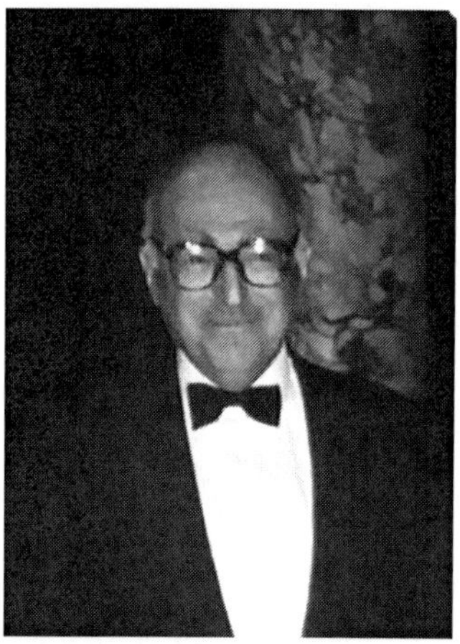

Dr. Kenneth Wormsley
(Photo: private)

It seemed curious to me that animal studies should have no impact on the clinical use of these types of drugs considering that humans and rats are more than 90% genetically identical.

The British doctor, Kenneth Wormsley, stated that omeprazole (the first proton pump inhibitor) is the first compound that has been accepted for clinical use after inducing cancer in its target organ in animal studies (Penston and Wormsley 1992). Therefore, the acceptance of omeprazole for clinical use broke a taboo.

Omeprazole was initially only used for severe ulcer disease, but gradually PPIs are now among the most frequently used drugs, and they are even regarded to be so harmless that they are able to be sold over the counter.

Despite the limited financial support locally, nationally, and from the European Union, we have been able to continue our research based on our knowledge of physiology and pathology using our patients and the local infrastructure. My collaborators' dedication has made it possible to perform research of a high standard with little money. It has been satisfying to see how many of our results, which were heavily disputed when first presented, are now gradually becoming accepted.

During all of these years of research within the same field, I have met a lot of resistance but I have also lived a good life. Medicine and science have taken me all over the world, and I have met some very interesting people. I got to know Nobel Laureate Sir James Black (Black et al. 1972), who even at his late age came to my 60th birthday party. He was a very nice man, and we liked each other. We often sat together sipping whiskey. He was the first to understand how to make new drugs by slightly changing the natural ligand so that it binds to, but does not elicit a response from, the actual receptor. This idea enabled him to make the first β-blocker propranolol and then, 7 years later, the first histamine-2 blocker, cimetidine.

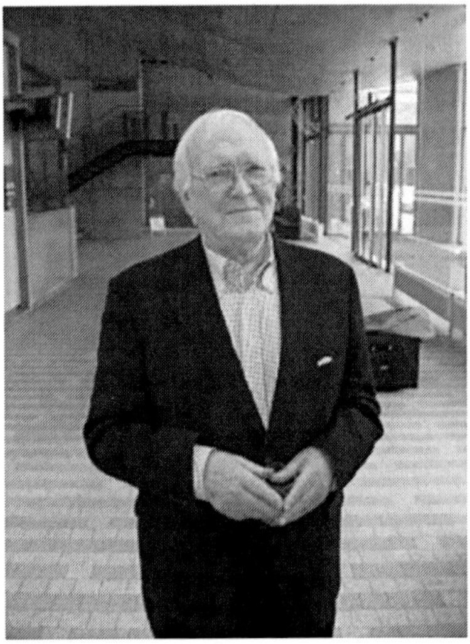

Nobel Laureate Sir James Black (Photo: private)

I would also like to mention Professor Irvin Modlin from Yale (Modlin, Bloom, and Mitchell 1979). I have known him for at least 20 years. He has sometimes supported me and sometimes turned me down, but he is the only American that has included me.

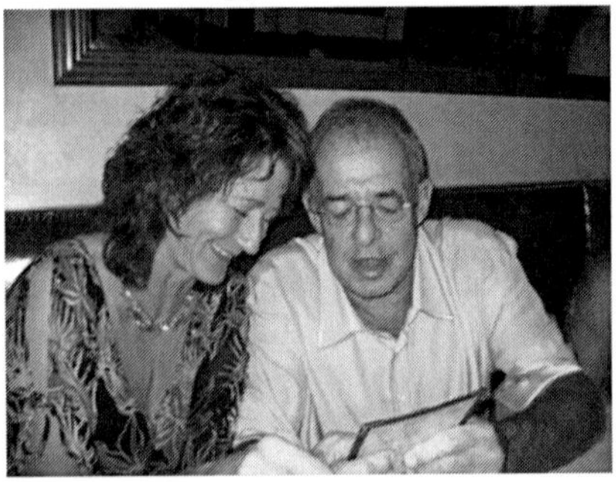

Professor Irvin Modlin with my wife (Photo: private)

When I started in medicine and science, I thought that colleagues supported each other. I was sad to realize that most people choose money over their colleagues. Over time I have learned to accept this. However,

I have often noticed rich but sad scientists because joy in science depends on freedom. Throughout my long career, I have seen how pharmaceutical companies control my field of medicine, and I suppose that it is similar in other areas. Few have had the opportunity to work and stay at the top of a very competitive area and I am very grateful that I was able to experience this.

I hope that the reader finds this book interesting. My experience is that evidence-based medicine, which is now so popular that it has become a mantra, is only studied for a short time, despite the fact that long-term side effects are possible. Animal toxicity studies should be given much more consideration than they are currently granted. Also, when toxic changes occur, the onus should be on the drug producer to convincingly demonstrate that there are qualitative differences between animals and man, which make animal experiments irrelevant.

It is a sad fact that directors and shareholders have received payments long before late but foreseen side effects are recognized. Throughout my career, the pharmaceutical industry has tried to stop me in different ways on various occasions. My experience is in gastroenterology, but I suppose it is the same in other areas of medicine. I hope that my experiences will be of general interest to the medical community, administrators, patients, and the general population.

References

Black, J. W., W. A. Duncan, C. J. Durant, C. R. Ganellin, and E. M. Parsons. 1972. "Definition and antagonism of histamine H 2 -receptors." *Nature* 236 (5347): 385-90. https://doi.org/10.1038/236385a0.

Bonfils, S., M. Mignon, and J. P. Accary. 1975. "Proceedings: Secretin provocation test in Zollinger-Ellison syndrome (Z.E.S.) with medical (metiamide) and/or surgical treatment." *Acta Hepatogastroenterol (Stuttg)* 22 (1): 60.

Burhol, P. G., T. G. Jenssen, I. Lygren, T. B. Schulz, R. Jorde, and H. L. Waldum. 1982. "Iodination with Iodo-gen and radioimmunoassay of cholecystokinin (CCK) in acidified plasma, CCK release, and molecular CCK components in man." *Digestion* 23 (3): 156-68. https://doi.org/10.1159/000198723.

Kleveland, P. M., S. E. Haugen, S. Sandvik, and H. L. Waldum. 1986. "The effect of pentagastrin on the gastric secretion by the totally isolated vascularly perfused rat stomach." *Scand J Gastroenterol* 21 (3): 379-84. https://doi.org/10.3109/00365528609003091.

Modlin, I. M., S. R. Bloom, and S. Mitchell. 1979. "VIP and the WDHA syndrome." *Gastroenterology* 76 (5 Pt 1): 1078-9.

Penston, J. G., and K. G. Wormsley. 1992. "Review article: maintenance treatment with H2-receptor antagonists for peptic ulcer disease."

Aliment Pharmacol Ther 6 (1): 3-29. https://doi.org/10.1111/j.1365-2036.1992.tb00541.x.

Petersen, H. 1969. "The relationship between the gastric and pancreatic secretion in man." *ScandJ Gastroenterol* 4 (4): 345-51. https://doi.org/10.3109/00365526909180615.

Rehfeld, J. F. 1973. "Gastrins in serum. A review of gastrin radioimmunoanalysis and the discovery of gastrin heterogeneity in serum." *Scand J Gastroenterol* 8 (7): 577-83.

von Houwelingen, R., A. Nordoy, E. van der Beek, U. Houtsmuller, M. de Metz, and G. Hornstra. 1987. "Effect of a moderate fish intake on blood pressure, bleeding time, hematology, and clinical chemistry in healthy males." *Am J Clin Nutr* 46 (3): 424-36. https://doi.org/10.1093/ajcn/46.3.424.

CHAPTER 2

GASTRIC JUICE AND ITS FUNCTION

Abstract

Gastric juice is a unique combination of a strong acid and active enzymes for the degradation of proteins (pepsin) and fat (lipase). This allows it to perform its main function of killing swallowed microorganisms. The production of acid in the upper part of the gastrointestinal tract was developed in primitive fish and this process has been preserved during evolution. Gastric acidity is tightly regulated by nerves (vagal nerves) and hormones (gastrin). Symptoms from the upper gastrointestinal tract are often accompanied by gastric acidic reflux. Therefore, patients, as well as doctors, have been interested in the regulation of gastric acid secretion. This process was among the first to be studied by Pavlov, who was famous for using experimental animal physiology (Pavlov 1902), demonstrating the importance of the vagal nerves. In the same period the hormonal concept was introduced (Bayliss & Starling, 1903). Shortly afterwards, Edkins (1906) postulated the presence of gastrin, which is produced by the G cell in the antral mucosa and released by proteins and the reduction of gastric acidity, reaches the acid production oxyntic mucosa via the blood. In 1920, Popielski showed that histamine was an efficient stimulator of acid secretion, which led to the discovery of the three principal gastric acid secretagogues: acetylcholine, gastrin, and histamine. However, their interaction, as well as the histamine-producing cell's part in the regulation, was disputed for decades. Gregory and Tracy purified and sequenced gastrin, while Berglindh and Öbrink developed the radioactive aminopyrine method to assess gastric acid secretion in isolated oxyntic glands and parietal cells. They showed that in contrast to histamine or a cholinergic agent, gastrin had no direct effect on rabbit glands or parietal cells. However, Soll's demonstration of gastrin's faint and inconsistent effect on similar canine preparations was given more credibility. We were able to unequivocally show that the gastrin receptor was on the histamine producing ECL cell and not on the parietal cell using an isolated rat's stomach.

In the middle of the eighties, Marshall and Warren showed that Helicobacter pylori caused chronic gastritis and peptic ulcer disease, which changed the focus on upper gastrointestinal diseases.

Keywords: acetylcholine; acid; ECL cell; function of gastrin; gastrin receptor; gastritis; Helicobacter pylori; histamine; parietal cell; peptic ulcer disease; regulation of gastric acid secretion.

The regulation of gastric acid secretion

In many ways, modern physiology began by studying the regulation of acid secretion, which reflects the significant interest that both clinicians and the general public have in gastric acidity.

Beaumont studied the regulation of gastric acid secretion in detail in a patient, who suffered from a gastric fistula, which was secondary to a shot accident, in the first half of the nineteenth century (Beaumont 1833). This single patient allowed him to perform studies and obtain results, which were later confirmed.

At the turn of the century, Bayliss and Starling (Bayliss and Starling 1903) created the hormone concept based upon studies centred on the secretion of water and bicarbonate from a denervated pancreas (secretin) and, a few years later, Edkins (1906) postulated the presence of a hormone which regulates gastric acidity produced in the stomach's antral mucosa (gastrin) (Edkins 1906). During the same period, in St. Petersburg, Pavlov started to use live animals (dogs) in his physiological research, which showed the importance of the vagal nerves in the stimulation of gastric acid secretion (Pavlov 1902).

More than a decade later, Popielski stated that histamine, a signal substance present in primitive animals as well as plants, also stimulated gastric acid secretion (Popielski 1920). Therefore, the three principal stimulators (secretagogues) of gastric acid secretion have been known for nearly a century. Their interactions were, however, disputed for more than fifty years.

Another disputed topic was the histamine-producing cell, which takes part in the regulation of gastric acid secretion. For a long time, the mast cell was the only cell in the acid producing gastric mucosa shown to produce histamine; this means it was thought to be the histamine source for the regulation of acid secretion. However, the mast cell has no fixed position with respect to the acid producing parietal cell, which would usually be expected for a regulatory cell.

In the late sixties in Lund, Håkanson described that a neuroendocrine rodent cell in gastric acid secreting mucosa also produced histamine. Due to the fact that it resembled the serotonin producing cell in the small intestine (the enterochromaffin cell) he named it the enterochromaffin-like cell (ECL) (Hakanson and Owman 1967).

During the same period in Lund, Kahlsson showed that meals and gastrin, which had recently been purified, sequenced, and synthesized by Gregory and Tracy (Gregory and Tracy 1961), released histamine and stimulated histamine synthesis in rodents (Kahlson et al. 1964). Nevertheless, American researchers believed that the mast cell produced the histamine and thus had a central role in the regulation of acid secretion in man.

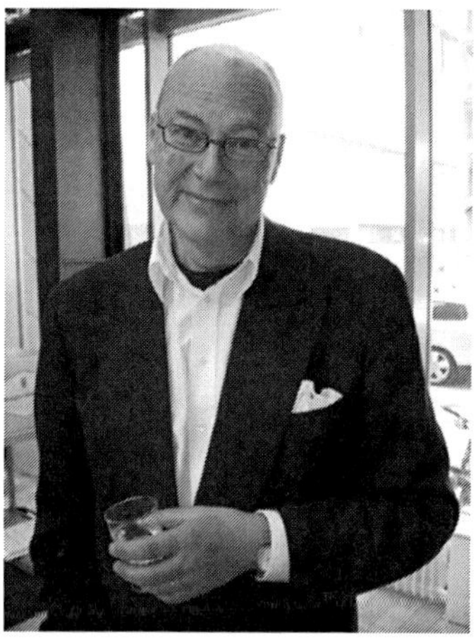

Professor Rolf Håkansson
(Photo: private)

Even after the Swedes, Berglindh et al. (Berglindh, Helander, and Obrink 1976) developed their method to study acid secretion in isolated glands and parietal cells via the accumulation of radioactively-labelled aminopyrine in the acid compartment and found no effect from gastrin, most scientists still believed that it had a direct stimulatory effect on the parietal cell. In fact, as late as 1997, the scientific community had not realized the physiological, and therefore the clinical, consequences of this new understanding of the regulation of gastric acid secretion.

Based upon our experiments on isolated rat stomach it was evident that gastrin works by releasing histamine from the ECL cell (Sandvik and Waldum 1991), and that the magnitude of the histamine release was a restrictive factor in gastrin stimulated acid secretion (Waldum, Lehy, et al. 1991). However, cholinergic stimulation was due to a direct effect on the parietal cell (Kleveland, Waldum, and Larsson 1987). Therefore, gastrin stimulated acid secretion does not give the maximum acid secretion. We explored this by combining gastrin stimulation with controlled (glucose clamp) hypoglycaemia through the stimulus of the vagal nerves, and we found, as expected, that the combined stimulation exceeded the effect from pentagastrin stimulation (Qvigstad et al. 1999). This study was also met with negativity and its findings were denied despite their accuracy.

Acid related diseases

It is well-known that gastric acid plays a central role in the pathogenesis of peptic ulcer disease. Therefore, before drugs became available, surgical methods were used to reduce acid secretion. These procedures could be debilitating and even lethal. Acid secretion could be reduced by removing the antrum of the stomach, which is where most of the gastrin producing G cells are located, or by removing the vagal nerves of the oxyntic mucosa (which is also called the parietal cell vagotomy). These operations are now rare because we have efficient drugs that are able to reduce gastric acid secretion. In addition, Marshall and Warren have proved that peptic ulcers are caused by Helicobacter pylori (Marshall and Warren 1984), which can be treated with antibiotics.

Besides peptic ulcer disease, gastric acid has a dominating role in the pathogenesis of gastro-oesophageal reflux disease (GERD). The oesophagus mucosa cannot withstand exposure to acidic gastric juice for a long time. Reflux does not only cause pain, but it also leads to inflammation with ulceration, which may cause fibrosis and stricture when it heals and, in the long-term, even predispose the sufferer to the risk of cancer. There has been a peculiar increase in GERD (Richter and Rubenstein 2018), which may be due to a reduction in the occurrence of Helicobacter pylori gastritis with reduced acid secretory capacity, or due to rebound acid hypersecretion secondary to the use of potent acid secretion inhibitors (Waldum et al. 1996). Furthermore, the increased numbers of overweight people have also probably contributed to the increased occurrence of GERD. The frequent

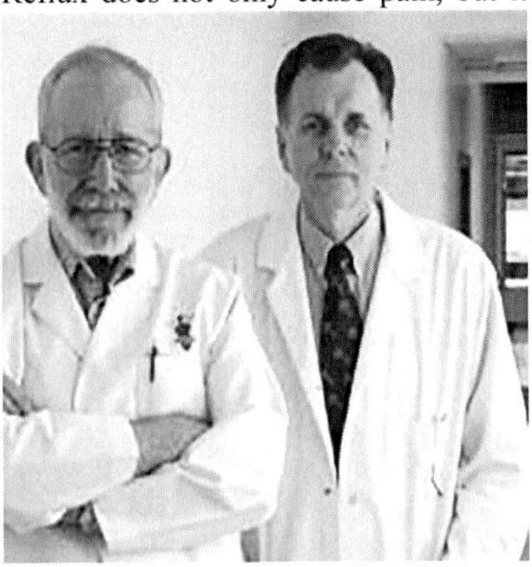

Nobel Prize Laureates Warren and Marshall
(Photo: By permission of the University of Western Australia)

occurrence of GERD has contributed to an increased usage of acid secretion inhibitors. The most efficient are proton pump inhibitors (PPIs), which are available over the counter. Therefore, many people have to live without normal functioning gastric juices, which may have long-term consequences.

Gastric juice is a unique combination of a strong acid and active enzymes, which degrade proteins (pepsin) and fat (lipase); however, its main function is killing swallowed microorganisms (Martinsen, Bergh, and Waldum 2005). The production of acid in the upper part of the gastrointestinal tract was first developed in primitive fish and this process has been preserved during evolution. Individually, gastric acidity is tightly regulated by the nerves (vagal nerves) and hormones (gastrin). Symptoms from the upper gastrointestinal tract are often accompanied by gastric acidic reflux. Therefore, patients as well as doctors have been interested in the regulation of gastric acid secretion. This process was among the first to be studied by Pavlov, who was famous for using experimental animal physiology (Pavlov 1902).demonstrating the important role of the vagal nerves. At the same time period Bayliss and Starling established the hormonal concept (Bayliss and Starling 1903), and Edkins postulated the presence of gastrin (Edkins 1906). Gastrin is produced by the G cell in the antral mucosa and released by proteins and the reduction of gastric acidity, reaches the acid production oxyntic mucosa via the blood. In 1920, Popielski showed that histamine was an efficient stimulator of acid secretion (Popielski 1920), which lead to the discovery of the three principal gastric acid secretagogues: acetylcholine, gastrin, and histamine. However, this interaction, as well as the histamine-producing cell's part in the regulation, was disputed for decades. Using the radioactive aminopyrine method to assess gastric acid secretion in isolated oxyntic glands and parietal cells, it was shown that gastrin, in contrast to histamine or a cholinergic agent, had no direct effect on rabbit glands/parietal cells (Berglindh, Helander, and Obrink 1976). However, Soll created a faint and inconsistent effect using gastrin on similar canine preparations (Soll 1982), which was considered to be more credible. It was possible to unequivocally show that the gastrin receptor was on the histamine producing ECL cell and not on the parietal cell using an isolated rat stomach (Waldum, Sandvik, et al. 1991; Bakke et al. 2001).

In the middle of the eighties, Marshall and Warren showed that Helicobacter pylori caused chronic gastritis and peptic ulcer disease (Marshall and Warren 1984). This changed the focus on upper gastrointestinal diseases.

References

Bakke, I., G. Qvigstad, A. K. Sandvik, and H. L. Waldum. 2001. "The CCK-2 receptor is located on the ECL cell, but not on the parietal cell." *Scand J Gastroenterol* 36 (11): 1128-33.

Bayliss, W. M., and E. H. Starling. 1903. "On the uniformity of the pancreatic mechanism in vertebrata." *J Physiol* 29 (2): 174-80. https://doi.org/10.1113/jphysiol.1903.sp000948.

Beaumont, W. 1833. *Experiments and obervation on the gastric juice and the physiology of digestion*. Plattsburg: Allen.

Berglindh, T., H. F. Helander, and K. J. Obrink. 1976. "Effects of secretagogues on oxygen consumption, aminopyrine accumulation and morphology in isolated gastric glands." *Acta Physiol Scand* 97 (4): 401-14. https://doi.org/10.1111/j.1748-1716.1976.tb10281.x.

Edkins, J. S. 1906. "The chemical mechanism of gastric secretion." *J Physiol* 34 (1-2): 133-44. https://doi.org/10.1113/jphysiol.1906.sp001146.

Gregory, R. A., and H. J. Tracy. 1961. "The preparation and properties of gastrin." *J Physiol* 156: 523-43. https://doi.org/10.1113/jphysiol.1961.sp006691.

Hakanson, R., and C. Owman. 1967. "Concomitant histochemical demonstration of histamine and catecholamines in enterochromaffin-like cells of gastric mucosa." *Life Sci* 6 (7): 759-66. https://doi.org/10.1016/0024-3205(67)90133-6.

Kahlson, G., E. Rosengren, D. Svahn, and R. Thunberg. 1964. "MOBILIZATION AND FORMATION OF HISTAMINE IN THE GASTRIC MUCOSA AS RELATED TO ACID SECRETION." *J Physiol* 174: 400-16.

Kleveland, P. M., H. L. Waldum, and H. Larsson. 1987. "Gastric acid secretion in the totally isolated, vascularly perfused rat stomach. A selective muscarinic-1 agent does, whereas gastrin does not, augment maximal histamine-stimulated acid secretion." *Scand J Gastroenterol* 22 (6): 705-13. https://doi.org/10.3109/00365528709011147.

Marshall, B. J., and J. R. Warren. 1984. "Unidentified curved bacilli in the stomach of patients with gastritis and peptic ulceration." *Lancet* 1 (8390): 1311-5.

Martinsen, T. C., K. Bergh, and H. L. Waldum. 2005. "Gastric juice: a barrier against infectious diseases." *Basic Clin Pharmacol Toxicol* 96 (2): 94-102. https://doi.org/10.1111/j.1742-7843.2005.pto960202.x.

Pavlov, I. 1902. The Work of the Digestive Glands. London Griffin.

Popielski, I. 1920. "β-Imidazolylyathyamin und die Organextracte Ester Teil." 178: 214-236.

Qvigstad, G., M. Bjorgaas, I. Eide, A. K. Sandvik, and H. L. Waldum. 1999. "Vagal stimulation augments maximal (penta) gastrin-stimulated acid secretion in humans." *Acta Physiol Scand* 165 (3): 277-81. https://doi.org/10.1046/j.1365-201x.1999.00514.x.

Richter, J. E., and J. H. Rubenstein. 2018. "Presentation and Epidemiology of Gastroesophageal Reflux Disease." *Gastroenterology* 154 (2): 267-276. https://doi.org/10.1053/j.gastro.2017.07.045.

Sandvik, A. K., and H. L. Waldum. 1991. "CCK-B (gastrin) receptor regulates gastric histamine release and acid secretion." *Am J Physiol* 260 (6 Pt 1): G925-8. https://doi.org/10.1152/ajpgi.1991.260.6.G925.

Soll, A. H. 1982. "Potentiating interactions of gastric stimulants on [14 C] aminopyrine accumulation by isolated canine parietal cells." *Gastroenterology* 83 (1 Pt 2): 216-23.

Waldum, H. L., J. S. Arnestad, E. Brenna, I. Eide, U. Syversen, and A. K. Sandvik. 1996. "Marked increase in gastric acid secretory capacity after omeprazole treatment." *Gut* 39 (5): 649-53.

Waldum, H. L., T. Lehy, E. Brenna, A. K. Sandvik, H. Petersen, B. S. Sognen, S. Bonfils, and M. J. Lewin. 1991. "Effect of the histamine-1 antagonist astemizole alone or with omeprazole on rat gastric mucosa." *Scand J Gastroenterol* 26 (1): 23-35.

Waldum, H. L., A. K. Sandvik, E. Brenna, and H. Petersen. 1991. "Gastrin-histamine sequence in the regulation of gastric acid secretion." *Gut* 32 (6): 698-701.

CHAPTER 3

PERSONAL CONTRIBUTIONS

Abstract

I began my work in Tromsø in the middle of the seventies with radioimmunoassays of gastrointestinal hormones and enzymes (pepsinogen I). I concentrated on gastric physiology. When I moved to Trondheim in 1981, the interaction between the three major gastric acid secretagogues—acetylcholine, gastrin, and histamine—was disputed. The available methods for studying the interaction were either too complex (studies in man and living animals) or too artificial, such as research on key enzymes (histidine decarboxylase). An isolated stomach model seemed ideal, but curiously it did not produce acid. However, the arterial perfusate used did not contain red blood cells, and the production of gastric acid lead to a concentration gradient of 1 million, which requires a lot of energy. Therefore, we added red blood cells to the perfusate and, when we applied a membrane oxygenator, the isolated rat stomach produced acid. This model allows us to have complete control over what goes into the stomach via both the vascular and luminal sides. It also allows us to collect both luminal and vascular effluents. Shortly afterwards we came across a sensitive and specific commercial immunoassay for histamine. By histamine determination in the vascular and acid titration in the luminal effluent we could show that the functional gastrin receptor was localized to the ECL cell. The idea that pentagastrin stimulated the maximal acid secretion was challenged, and it was shown that maximal acid secretion depended on both the ECL cell and parietal cell masses, which explains why profound acid inhibition with proton pump inhibitors (PPIs) induced rebound acid inhibition. Combining vagal stimulation by controlled hypoglycemia using a glucose-clamp and the maximum effect dose of pentagastrin also increased acid secretion beyond the amount produced by pentagastrin alone. In rat studies, we showed that a positive trophic of gastrin on the ECL cell followed the same concentration dependence as the functional one and reached the maximum at a lower level than previously realized. Consequently, we began to study the ECL cell's role in gastric carcinomas and eventually proved that ECL cell differentiation in cancer cells occurred in a portion of the carcinomas, particularly in the diffuse type and the signet ring subtype. All of these studies were difficult to get published and were generally negatively received. Moreover, most "experts" in the field never mentioned them.

Keywords: acid; classification of carcinomas; ECL cell; gastric cancer; gastrin; gastrin receptor; histamine; interactions between secretagogues; maximal gastric acid secretion; parietal cell; rebound acid hypersecretion; regulation of gastric acid secretion.

The acid producing isolated rat's stomach

When we started to study the role of gastrin in gastric carcinogenesis in the early eighties in Trondheim, it became apparent that there was a need for a new method of assessing biological gastrin activity. Studying the regulation of acid secretion in humans or in awake or anesthetized animals requires complex models, whereas studies on isolated parietal cells or oxyntic glands could give false results due to the risk of damage to receptors or other key molecules during preparation.

An isolated stomach artificially perfused through the lumen and the vascular bed without recirculation looked like a promising compromise. However, at that time, nobody had succeeded in making an isolated stomach produce acid. Previous attempts at establishing a model to perform this function used oxygenated buffers to perfuse the vascular bed.

Taking into consideration that stomach acid production probably requires the most energy in the body, which creates a concentration gradient of more than one million H+, it appeared that the lack of acid secretion could be due to O_2 deficiency. We started to first add human red cells to the buffer and then O_2 by bubbling; however, this was not successful. Then we contacted engineers who were working with membrane oxygenators at our university's technology faculty. At the same time, Short et al. reported success when using ovine red cells in this procedure (Short, Wolfe, and McGuigan 1984). We then succeeded in creating a stable reproducible model to study the regulation of acid secretion, which allowed a comparison between the release of mediators to the blood and the secretion of acid to the lumen (Kleveland, Haugen, and Waldum 1986). This model was in use over a fifteen years period in our laboratory. Previously, it had been an accepted fact that maximal gastric acid secretion could be induced by stimulation with either histamine or gastrin.

Due to histamine's general toxicity, it has to be given with a histamine-1-antagonist (Kay 1953) or alternatively use a selective histamine-2 agonist (Durant et al. 1978). However, even when histamine was given with a histamine-1 antagonist, there was some toxicity preventing a further increase to the histamine dose. Furthermore, it was not proven that the histamine agonists, such as impromidine, were complete histamine-2 agonists. Therefore, maximal gastric acid secretion during histamine stimulation in humans and living animals has not yet been completely explored; this means that the belief that maximal gastrin and histamine stimulated acid secretions are similar has not been experimentally proven.

With the isolated rat stomach, we could soon show that the maximal histamine stimulated acid secretion exceeded that of gastrin (Kleveland, Waldum, and Larsson 1987). Furthermore, gastrin did not have any additive stimulatory effect on maximal histamine stimulated acid secretion, which is in contrast to a cholinergic agent. These findings clearly showed that gastrin stimulated acid secretion through the stimulation of histamine, which obviously was a restrictive factor in terms of gastrin stimulated, and therefore meal stimulated, acid secretion.

Maximal gastric acid secretion in man

This new physiological insight has great clinical implications, as exemplified by rebound acid hypersecretion after the long-term inhibition of acid secretion (Waldum, Arnestad, et al. 1996). Moreover, we were also able to show that vagal stimulation augmented maximal gastrin stimulated acid secretion in humans (Qvigstad, Bjorgaas, et al. 1999). Therefore, gastrin stimulated acid secretion is an imperfect parameter for maximal gastric acid secretion (Waldum, Brenna, and Sandvik 1998).

This new concept was met with negative attitudes, as shown in the following correspondence with *Gastroenterology*.

Gastroenterology
Official Journal of the American Gastroenterological Association

7910 Woodmont Avenue, 7th Floor
Bethesda, MD 20814-3015
Phone: 301 / 941-9781 • Fax: 301 / 951-0757

October 29, 1997

FAX: 47 (73)997546

Helge L. Waldum, M.D.
Trondheim University Hospital
Department of Medicine
Univ I Trondheim
N-7006 Trondheim
NORWAY

RE: Manuscript No. 97-7576-00

Dear Dr. Waldum:

We regret to inform you that your manuscript entitled "Maximal Gastric Acid Secretion In Man - A Concept That Needs Precision" was not accepted for publication in *Gastroenterology*. The manuscript was assessed by two reviewers, the Associate Editor, and the Board of Editors. Both reviewers acknowledged the interest of this study but also pointed out several shortcomings, as can be seen in the copies attached. Important criticism related to the need for a test and the lack of convincing proof in favor of the test proposed. Because of these limitations, we were unable to assign a publishable priority to this manuscript.

We regret that these concerns preclude publication in *Gastroenterology*, but we hope you find the enclosed comments of the reviewer(s) useful when submitting your paper to another journal. We look forward to future submissions of other manuscripts.

Sincerely,

Guido N.J. Tytgat, ~~M.D.~~
Associate Editor

Daniel K. Podolsky, M.D.
Editor

Reviewer A Manuscript No. 97-7576-00 Date 10/1/97

SPECIFIC

PAGE	PARA	
3	3	Is the ECL cell the principal histamine-producing and -releasing cell in all species?
4	1	The authors imply that Dr. Kopin and colleagues actually may have cloned the gastrin receptor from ECL cell contaminants in their canine parietal cell preparation. Have they carefully examined those elegant studies? Moreover, do they also attribute the findings of Dr. Soll and colleagues to contamination? Both of these investigators did indeed use "very" (not "wery") pure cell preparations, and owing to marked differences in cell density, it is likely that any contamination occurred from mucus, and not ECL, cells.

GASTROENTEROLOGY

Reviewer A Manuscript No. 97-7576-00 Date 10/1/97

REVIEWER'S COMMENTS TO AUTHORS

GENERAL

This manuscript by Professor Waldum and colleagues attempts to provide a new definition for maximal acid secretion in humans. While the concept is sound, in too many instances, the authors cross species and extrapolate results. Furthermore, many of the new methods recommended have not been adequately validated in humans. Finally, a rationale for the need to measure maximal acid output in the clinical arena in present day medicine has not been provided.

Reviewer B Manuscript No. 97-7576-00 Date 10/8/97

SPECIFIC

PAGE	PARA	
4	1	There is overwhelming data from numerous sources supporting the conclusion that there is a CCK_B receptor on parietal cells. To leave the reader with the implication this is not so, seems an inappropriate conclusion.

Specific Points:

1. There are numerous misspelled words and the manuscript should be carefully proofread.

2. Reference 44 lacks a title.

GASTROENTEROLOGY

Reviewer B Manuscript No. 97-7576-00 Date 10/8/97

REVIEWER'S COMMENTS TO AUTHORS

GENERAL

This is an interesting study but it has two major weaknesses:

a. First, the author does not clearly make the case why such a test is needed. In what clinical conditions or situations would it be needed? Even more important, does it really add anything to existing tests? For example, if current methods measure 90% of maximal secretion and the result is primarily proportional to parietal cell mass in most patients, why do we need another test?

b. Second, *in vitro* the evidence the author presents, that pentagastrin alone does not give a maximal response, is relatively convincing. However, *in vivo*, with variable basal histamine secretion and cholinergic tone, the data is much less convincing. Furthermore, the difference from absolute maximum may be very small.

NTNU - NORGES TEKNISK-NATURVITENSKAPELIGE UNIVERSITET
DET MEDISINSKE FAKULTET
MEDISINSK AVDELING
REGIONSYKEHUSET I TRONDHEIM

TELEFAX

Appeal to the editors of Gastroenterology 1997

Til/To: GASTROENTEROLOGY
Attn.: Editor Daniel K. Podolsky
Telefax: 1 301 951-0757

Dato/Date: 12.11.97

Fra/From: Professor Helge L. Waldum
Telefax: 73 99 75 46

Antall sider inkludert denne:
(Number of pages including this)

Hvis du ikke mottar alle sidene, vennligst ring Berit Myren, 73 99 85 60. (In case you do not receive all pages, please call Berit Myren+ 47).

Melding/Message

Re: Manuscript No. 97-7576-00

Dear Editor Daniel K. Podolsky,

Thank you for your comments on our manuscript concerning maximal acid secretion in man. Of course, I was sorry to find so much criticism and learning that the manuscript was rejected. On the other hand, this was not surprising since we have sent many manuscripts to your journal previously which have been rejected although the results and concepts have been confirmed many years later. Concerning the comments by the reviewers and by the Editorial Board, I will make the following remarks:

We have not argued for a new test to be used routinely for assessing maximal acid secretion. However, it still is important to measure acid secretion in clinical research as confirmed by our recent finding of increased maximal gastric secretion after stopping treatment with proton pump inhibitors (Gut 1996; 39: 649-653). Initially we had problems in having that manuscript accepted because the reviewers did not understand that the ECL cell mass is a critical factor for maximal gastrin stimulated acid secretion. That paper actually proves that also in man the ECL cell plays a central role in the regulation of gastric acid secretion. Furthermore, it was quite surprising that your reviewers still localize the CCK-B receptor to the parietal cell. After all, Gastroenterology had a front cover figure (March 1996) where the gastrin receptor was localized to the ECL cell. Actually that front figure was commented on by our group because the original figure was published first by us in 1991 (Gut 1991; 33: 698-701), although your journal referred to other and later references. Our letter was printed in Gastroenterology 1996; 111: 838-839.

Taking into consideration that Gastroenterology had used a figure on the front page with the gastrin/CCK B receptor only on the ECL cell, I find it hard to understand that it should be too provocative to claim that the functional important gastrin receptor is localized to the ECL cell.

UNIVERSITETET I TRONDHEIM

The other point made by both reviewers is that they do not see any need for a test for maximal gastric acid secretion in clinical use. Moreover, rewiever A argues that we are crossing species and extrapolating results. What about the study of Kopin et al., which was done on canine mucosal cells (Proc Nat Acad Sci USA 1992; 89: 3605-9)? Moreover, even in the dog it has been convincingly demonstrated that gastrin releases histamine showing that even in that species a functionally important gastrin receptor is localized to the ECL cell (J Pharmacol Exp Ther;1987:243:887-92). We have previously thoroughly discussed the question of species differences with regard to the regulation of gastric acid secretion (Gastrin: histamine releasing activity, page 259-71. In: Gastrin. JH Walsh (ed). Raven press 1993).

I was very surprised to find that a rewiever of Gastroenterology indirectly claims that the mast cell plays a role in the regulation of gastric acid secretion. It was convinsingly shown many years ago, that the mast cell histamine is unrelated to the acid secretory process. The view point by your reviewer is hopelessly outdated.

The studies of Soll in the early eighties, although very important at time, were probably misinterpreted with regard to the localization of the gastrin receptor. His results are best explained by gastrin releasing histamine from ECL cells, and that this released histamine secondarily stimulates nearby parietal cells explaining the slight stimulatory effect on aminopyrine uptake by gastrin (Am J Physiol 1980;238: G366-75). I was surprised to learn that the Editorial Board of Gastroenterology and both your reviewers did not find it important to know and determine maximal gastric acid secretory capacity. It should be recalled that a correct understanding of the physiological regulation of gastric acid secretion is necessary to explain the acid hypersecretion provoked by hypergastrinemia whether induced by inhibitors of gastric acid secretion (Gut 1996; 39: 649-53) or by gastrinomas, and especially a rapid fall in maximal acid secretion after radical surgery for gastrinomas (Gastroenterology 1992;102:776-8). We did not advocate that gastric acid secretion should be determined in an everyday clinical setting, but it is nevertheless important for experts and gastroenterologists to have a correct knowledge of gastric physiology, not least to understand the side-effects of drugs. In this context I must add that I am worried to see that journals easily accept manuscripts showing no danger or important side-effects by inhibitors of gastric acid secretion, while it is always very difficult to get a manuscript focusing on negative effects, accepted. In an indirect way also our manuscript focuses of the functional consequences of inhibition of gastric acid secretion.

If you find the arguments above of interest and of importance, we could change the manuscript in order to avoid misinterpretations. Particularly, a chapter on the indications for the determination of gastric acid secretion could be added, and the presence of the gastrin receptor on the ECL cell and not on the parietal cell could be changed to: The functional important gastrin receptor is localized in the ECL cell.

I hope for an answer in the near future.

Sincerely yours

Helge L. Waldum
Professor of Medicine

Gastroenterology

Official Journal of the American Gastroenterological Association

7910 Woodmont Avenue, 7th Floor
Bethesda, MD 20814-3015
Phone: 301 / 941-9781 • Fax: 301 / 951-0757

December 16, 1997

Helge L. Waldum, M.D.
Trondheim University Hospital
Department of Medicine
Section of Gastroenterology
Univ I Trondheim
N-7006 Trondheim
NORWAY

RE: Manuscript No. 97-7576-01

Dear Dr. Waldum:

We have received your letter of appeal and once again re-examined your manuscript "Maximal Gastric Acid Secretion In Man - A Concept That Needs Precision" and its two reviews. Unfortunately, we must again inform you that your manuscript cannot be accepted for publication. We agree with many of the points raised in your appeal letter regarding the importance of the ECL cell. However, the crucial issues raised in the initial review of your manuscript centered on whether a new test(s) is really needed to measure maximal acid secretory capacity, and whether such a test has been rigorously studied and validated in human patients. While many of your ideas are quite interesting, *Gastroenterology* gives priority to manuscripts to original data from clinical or basic laboratory investigations. As such, your manuscript falls somewhat short, and thus we are unable to assign your manuscript a priority score sufficient for publication.

Sincerely,

Timothy Wang, M.D.
Associate Editor

Daniel K. Podolsky, M.D.
Editor

After being rejected by *Gastroenterology*, the manuscript showing that maximal gastrin stimulation does not represent maximal acid secretory capacity was sent to *Gut*. The Editor, Professor Farthing handled the manuscript fairly, but the reviewers came up with invalid arguments to block publication.

Gut

An International Journal of Gastroenterology and Hepatology

Published by the BMJ Publishing Group

BMA HOUSE
TAVISTOCK SQUARE
LONDON WC1H 9JR
International: +44 171 383 6157
Direct Line: 0171 383 6157
Fax: 0171 383 6787
E.Mail: gut_journal@compuserve.com
Website: www.gutjnl.com

24 April 1998

PROFESSOR HELGE L WALDUM
SECTION OF GASTROENTEROLOGY
UNIVERSITY HOSPITAL OF TRONDHEIM
N-7006 TRONDHEIM
NORWAY

Dear Professor Waldum

Re: GUT/1998/139 - *VAGAL STIMULATION AUGMENTS MAXIMAL (PENTA) GASTRIN STIMULATED ACID SECRETION IN MAN*

Thank you for submitting this paper to *Gut*, which was discussed at the last editorial committee meeting. I am sorry to say that I am unable to accept it for publication on this occasion and return your manuscript with regret. I am enclosing referees' comments; you may find them helpful if you wish to resubmit your manuscript to another journal.

Kind regards

Yours sincerely

Professor M J G Farthing
Editor

GUT

Sheet 2 **COMMENTS FOR AUTHORS**

Gut Ref No G98/139 (2)

This study shows that the peak value of acid outputs in healthy humans achieved by infusion of pentagastrin at a dose of 6 µg/kg-h can be significantly increased (by about 20%) by combining this pentagastrin infusion with insulin-induced hypoglycemia. This insulin-induced stimulation alone (without pentagastrin) applied with glucose-clamp technique produced relatively lower response than that achieved with pentagastrin alone.

General comments

1. It is not clear whether pentagastrin infused i.v. at a dose of 6 µg/kg-h really produced maximal acid secretion in these subjects. Dose-response to pentagastrin should be obtained rather than single dose administration of pentagastrin because such dose could lead to the fall in the blood pressure and to the discomfort-like nausea that is mentioned in Result section. I would like to see the dose-response to pentagastrin and then to pick up the maximal acid output to be used as maximal acid response to this secretagogue to be sure whether we really deal with the maximal acid secretory activity.

2. I do not understand why infusion of insulin with glucose clamp technique could not be carried out for longer time than 30 min to match time period of the infusion of pentagastrin. In fact, Fig. 1 shows that the peak acid response to insulin was not achieved during infusion of this secretagogue but much after the period of hypoglycemia. This 60 min insulin hypoglycemia could be more preferable way of stimulation of acid secretion than just 30 min. Again, to be sure that maximal acid response to insulin was achieved various doses of insulin should be applied.

3. The number of tested subjects (N = 8) is rather small so I would like to see individual data for acid output in each subject tested and the data should be expressed as medians and interquartile or full range.

This study shows that the peak value of acid output in healthy humans achieved by infusion of pentagastrin at a dose of 6 µg/kg-h can be significantly increased (by about 20%) by combining this pentagastrin infusion with insulin-induced hypoglycemia. This insulin-induced stimulation alone (without pentagastrin) applied with glucose-clamp technique produced relatively lower response than that achieved with pentagastrin alone.

General comments

1. It is not clear whether pentagastrin infused i.v. at a dose of 6µg/kg-h really produced maximal acid secretion in these subjects. Dose- response to pentagastrin should be obtained rather than single dose administration of pentagastrin because such dose could lead to the fall in the blood pressure

and to discomfort-like nauseas that is mentioned in Result section. I would like to see the dose-response to pentagastrin and then to pick up the maximal acid output to be used as maximal acid response to this secretagogue to be sure whether we really deal with the maximal acid secretory capacity.

2. I do not understand why infusion of insulin with glucose clamp technique could not be carried out for longer time than 30 min to match time period of the infusion of pentagastrin. In fact, Fig. 1 shows that the peak acid response to insulin was not achieved during infusion of this secretagogue but much after the period of hypoglycemia. This 60 min insulin hypoglycemia could be more preferable way of stimulation of acid secretion than just 30 min. Again, to be sure that maximal acid response to insulin was achieved various doses of insulin should be applied.

3. The number of tented subjects (N=8) is rather small so I would like to individual data for acid output in each subject tested and the data should be expressed as medians and interquartile or full range.

GUT

Sheet 2 **COMMENTS FOR AUTHORS**

Gut Ref No G98/139 (1)

The authors report a higher acid output when calculated as peak acid output in response to hypoglycaemia plus pentagastrin compared to that achieved with pentagastrin alone. In real terms, the difference is relatively small with the latter being 20% lower.

The results would have been more convincing if a difference had also been apparent when the results were analysed as maximal acid output rather than just peak acid output. This is especially the case when studies have been done on a relatively small number (8) subjects.

In addition, the results would have been more convincing if the pentagastrin alone studies had been repeated with an even higher dose of pentagastrin in order to ensure that the maximal response to pentagastrin was indeed being achieved.

NTNU
NORGES TEKNISK-NATURVITENSKAPELIGE UNIVERSITET

Editor Professor MJG Farthing
BMJ Publishing Group
BMA House Tavistock Square
London WC1H 9JR
ENGLAND

DET MEDISINSKE FAKULTET
Medisinsk avdeling
Gastroenterologisk seksjon

Vår saksbehandler:

Telefon:

Deres dato:	Deres ref.:	Vår dato:	Vår ref.:
		06-05-98	HLW/bm

Ref. Gut 1998/12 - Maximal gastric acid secretion in man. A concept that needs precision

Thank you for the evaluation of the above mentioned manuscript which, however, unfortunately was not accepted for publication in your journal.

This letter only to make you aware of that it was not at all obvious from the referee's report that it should be rejected since the reviewer stated that it was an interesting review and that he only had some concern concerning style of the manuscript which the reviewer indeed made contribution to improve. I am therefore unable to understand why the manuscript was not accepted for publication.

Re. Gut 1998/139 - Vagal stimulation augments maximal (penta) gastrin stimulated acid secretion in man

The above mentioned manuscript was also refused for publication in your journal. There I got a report from two reviewers. Both of these reports are surprisingly negative in attitude towards the work. None of them give us any credit for introducing a completely new technique in vagal stimulation (glucose clamp hypoglycaemia). It is also very depressing to see that referee no. 1 argues that it would have been much more convincing if the results have been analysed as maximal acid output and not just peak acid output. Peak acid output does of course represent the maximal acid secretory capacity of the gastric mucosa better than maximal acid output, since there for instance is a lag period before acid secretion increases when stimulated.

Moreover, it is stated that we studied a relatively small number (eight) subjects. I have always believed that statistics take into account the number of subjects studied?

The last section in the referee's comment is even more depressing since the concentration response curve for pentagastrin with respect to gastric acid secretion has been studied thoroughly by a large number of authors previously. I feel that it would not be justified and perhaps also unethical to repeat such a study where the results are so well available from literature.

Adresse/Address:
Regionsykehuset i Trondheim
N-7006 Trondheim
Norway

Editor. GUT. 06.05.

Norwegian University of Science and Technology
Faculty of Medicine
Department of Medicine
Section of Gastroenterology
Int. phone: + 47 73 99 86 60
Int. fax: + 47 73 99 75 46

Gut
An International Journal of Gastroenterology and Hepatology
Published by the BMJ Publishing Group

13 May 1998

BMA HOUSE
TAVISTOCK SQUARE
LONDON WC1H 9JR
International: +44 171 387 4499
Telephone: 0171 387 4499
Direct Line: 0171 383 6157
Fax: 0171 383 6787
E.mail: 101317.465@compuserve.com
Website: www.gutjnl.com

PROFESSOR HELGE L WALDUM
PROFESSOR OF MEDICINE
SECTION OF GASTROENTEROLOGY
NORWEGIAN UNIVERSITY OF SCIENCE
N-7006 TRONDHEIM
NORWAY

Dear Professor Waldum

Re: GUT/1998/139 - VAGAL STIMULATION AUGMENTS MAXIMAL (PENTA) GASTRIN STIMULATED ACID SECRETION IN MAN

Thank you for your letter about this manuscript, pointing out your concerns about the referees' reports. I shall send your letter to the reviewers and ask them for their specific omments on the points you raise. This, however, does not indicate the manuscript has renetered the appraisal system. I will write again as soon as I have their comments.

With kind regards.

Yours sincerely,

Professor M J G Farthing
Editor

Gut

An International Journal of Gastroenterology and Hepatology

Published by the BMJ Publishing Group

13 May 1998

BMA HOUSE
TAVISTOCK SQUARE
LONDON WC1H 9JR
International: +44 171 387 4499
Telephone: 0171 387 4499
Direct Line: 0171 383 6157
Fax: 0171 383 6787
E.mail: 101317.465@compuserve.com
Website: www.gutjnl.com

PROFESSOR HELGE L WALDUM
PROFESSOR OF MEDICINE
SECTION OF GASTROENTEROLOGY
NORWEGIAN UNIVERSITY OF SCIENCE
N-7006 TRONDHEIM
NORWAY

Dear Professor Waldum

Re: GUT/1998/12 - MAXIMAL GASTRIC ACID SECRETION IN MAN. A CONCEPT THAT NEEDS PRECISION

Your manuscript was reviewed by myself and the associate editors. We decided on the basis of our own assessment and that of external peer review, that the manuscript did not achieve a high enough priority score to enable us to publish the manuscript in *Gut*. Unfortunately, we receive about four times as many manuscripts as we are able to publish in the journal and this inevitably means that some worthy material must be rejected. I am sorry that your manuscript fell into this category on this occasion.

With kind regards.

Yours sincerely,

Professor M J G Farthing
Editor

05/08 '98 15:41 FAX 44 171 383 6787 GUT EDITORIAL 001

Gut

An International Journal of Gastroenterology and Hepatology

Published by the BMJ Publishing Group

BMA HOUSE
TAVISTOCK SQUARE
LONDON WC1H 9JR

International: +44 171 383 6157
Telephone: 0171 383 6157
0171 383 6394
Fax: 0171 383 6787
E.mail: gut_journal@compuserve.com
Website: www.gutjnl.com

COPY

27 July 1998

Professor Helge L Waldum
University Hospital of Trondheim
Department of Medicine
N-7005 Trondheim
Norway

Dear Professor Waldum

Re: GUT/1998/139 - Vagal stimulation augments maximal (penta) gastrin stimulated acid secretion in man

I returned your manuscript to both reviewers and I discussed their responses with the associate editors, at our recent editorial committee meeting. Both reviewers produced cogent arguments why they did not wish to move their ground and we felt, therefore, that we should adhere to our initial decision, to reject the manuscript. I am sorry to have to disappoint you on this occasion.

With kind regards.

Yours sincerely,

Professor M J G Farthing
Editor

15:41 FAX 44 171 383 6787 GUT EDITORIAL 002

G98/139 ①

GUT/1998/139 - VAGAL STIMULATION AUGMENTS MAXIMAL (PENTA) GASTRIN STIMULATED ACID SECRETION IN MAN.

I have read the authors' comments and do not believe that they invalidate the comments I made in my review. I still believe the results would have been more convincing if they had been seen in both the maximal acid output and peak acid output measurements. The authors have not satisfactorily explained why they were not apparent in the maximal acid output measurements. The authors criticised me for commenting about the relatively small numbers of subjects studied However, if they had taken the time to do more subjects, they might well have found significance with both the maximal acid output and peak acid output which would certainly have made the result much more robust.

I read carefully again the paper of Qvigstad et al entitled "Vagal
stimulation augments maximal (penta)gastrin stimulated acid secretion" and
found it equally unacceptable for the publication in Gut as its original
version.
My major concern is that it is not possible to determine whether
insulin hypoglycemia really augments maximal acid response to pentagastrin
using only single dose of each secretagogue (pentagastrin or insulin) was
used or in combination. According to my experience the maximal acid
response to pentagastrin infused i.v. could be achieved usually at much
lower than 6 μg/kg-h and and this response shows great individual
variations so the dose 6 μg/kg-h could be supramaximal resulting in the
fall of secretion after initial increase. Therefore, it seems necessary
first to obtain dose-response to each secretgogue alone and then
on separate day test to combine the peak response to each seretagogue to see
whether such combination results in further rise in gastric acid output.
I requested that the table with individual data for each of the
secretagogues at each time period tested should be included but this simple
presentation has not been done.
I agree with Authors that the use of glucose clamp technique to
maintain hypoglycemia seems novel in testing gastric secretion but, again, why
only one dose of insulin or one hypoglycemia level was used in attempt to
enhance maximal acid response to pentagastrin ?. The presentation only of
the glucose clamp hypoglycemia does not justify the publication of this
paper in gut.
Under these conditions, I believe that the paper adds very little to
our knowledge about gastric acid secretion in humans and do not think that
it could be considered suitable for the publication in Gut.

"I read carefully again the paper by Qvigstad et al entitled "Vagal stimulation augments maximal (penta)gastrin stimulated acid secretion" and found it equally unacceptable for the publication in Gut as its original version.

My major concern is that it is not possible to determine whether insulin hypoglycemia really augments maximal acid response to pentagastrin using only single dose of each secretagogue (pentagastrin or insulin) was used or in combination. According to my experiences the maximal acid response to pentagastrin infused i.v. could be achieved usually at much lower than 6 μg/kg-h and this response shows great individual variations so the dose 6 μg/kg-h could be supramaximal resulting in a fall of secretion after initial increase. Therefore, it seems necessary first to obtain dose-response to each secretagogue alone and then on separate day test to combine the peak response to each secretagogue to see whether such combination results in further rise in gastric acid output.

I requested that the table with individual data for each of the secretagogue at each time period tested should be included but this simple presentation has not been done.

I agree with the Authors that the use of glucose clamp technique to maintain hypoglycemia seems novel in testing gastric secretion but, again, why only one dose of insulin or one hypoglycemia level was used in the attempt to enhance maximal acid response to pentagastrin? The presentation only of the glucose clamp hypoglycemia does not justify does not justify the publication of this paper in gut.

Under these conditions, I believe that this paper adds very little to our knowledge about gastric acid secretion in humans and do not think that it should be considered suitable for publication in Gut."

It was hard to accept refusal based upon these reports. One of them asked for a dose response for insulin, as they were apparently unaware of how insulin stimulates acid secretion through threshold hypoglycemia. However, we were also asked why we did not prolong the insulin stimulation. Again, the reviewer was apparently unaware of the discomfort felt during hypoglycemia. All of the suggestions by the two reviewers at best indicated a lack of familiarity with acid secretory studies on humans or, at worst, fabricated arguments to prevent publication.

Both the study showing that vagal stimulation by hypoglycemia augmented maximal gastrin stimulated acid secretion (Qvigstad, Bjorgaas, et al. 1999) and a review on maximal gastric acid secretion (Waldum, Brenna, and Sandvik 1998) were eventually published. The findings in these papers, as well as the conclusions, have not been disputed, although it must be admitted that very few scientists and clinicians are interested in acid secretion anymore. It seems that the attitude is that gastric acidity is an old problem because we have PPIs to manage it.

Determination of histamine

In the isolated rat stomach model, both the vascular bed and the stomach lumen are perfused, which allows the collection of both vascular and luminal fluids for further analysis. Since the initial studies indirectly showed that gastrin worked by stimulating histamine release (Kleveland, Waldum, and Larsson 1987), it became mandatory to determine the levels of histamine in the venous liquid coming from the stomach. At that time, according to Lorenz, the fluorometric method was the most frequently used (Lorenz et al. 1991). However, this type of chemical method would be expected to be unspecific due to the interference from precursors and metabolites, as well as other related substances.

At that time, however, a French group succeeded in making a histamine radioimmunoassay (Morel and Delaage 1988). They produced antibodies against histamine coupled with albumin prior to analysis. There are two specific steps in this method: the albumin coupling and the antibody binding. The method is therefore rather specific and, like most immunoassays, sensitive (Waldum, Sandvik, et al. 1991). With this assay, we were able to show that gastrin elicited enough of an instantaneous concentration dependent histamine release to explain gastrin's acid stimulatory effect (Sandvik et al. 1987).

We felt that our findings had solved a dispute that had been ongoing for more than 60 years about the interaction of gastric acid secretagogues and the localization of the gastrin receptor. The manuscript was sent to *Gut*, but it was refused because we had applied a new method for the determination of histamine, which led one of the reviewers to believe that it had not been properly validated (Lorenz et al. 1991). This was the first, but not the last time, that important work has been refused due to scientists protecting their own research and findings. Of course, an immunoassay is *a priori* more specific than a chemical method. The manuscript was later published in another journal (Sandvik et al. 1987) and the findings are undisputed.

Studies on isolated oxyntic mucosal cells

There was obviously a discrepancy between the results by Berglindh et al. concerning the way gastrin works when stimulating acid secretion in isolated rabbit oxyntic cells (Berglindh, Helander, and Obrink 1976), as well as our work on an isolated rat's stomach (Kleveland, Waldum, and Larsson 1987; Sandvik et al. 1987), and Soll's studies (Soll 1982) on isolated gastric cells from dogs.

We repeated our studies on rat gastric cells where we concomitantly determined the effect of gastrin on acid secretion and on the histamine concentration in the medium (Brenna and Waldum 1991). We found an inconsistent effect from gastrin on acid secretion in isolated parietal cells but, interestingly, this only occurred in preparations where we found an increase in the histamine concentration in the medium. Our manuscript was rejected by *Acta Physiologica Scandinavica*, and initially also by the Scandinavian *Journal of Gastroenterology*, but it was accepted after direct contact with the editor of the latter journal. Curiously, a similar study was published a year later in *Gastroenterology* (Prinz et al. 1993) and was deemed to be so important that one of its illustrations was displayed on the front page of the journal. Interestingly, one of the authors of this study was from Sweden and possibly one of the reviewers for the two Scandinavian journals. *Gastroenterology* accepted a letter focusing on the localization of the gastrin receptor (Waldum, Sandvik, et al. 1996).

[...]SIOLOGICA SCANDINAVICA

Manuscript No. ....

[...] of paper: A comparison between the effects of histamine and pentagastrin on rat parietal cells. Pentagastrin stimulates aminopyridin uptake in isolated rat parietal cells by releasing histamine from the enterochromaffine like cells

Name of author(s): E. Brenna, A.K. Sandvik and H.L. Waldum

Referee,s comments for attention of authors:

In the manuscript 'A comparison between the effects of histamine and pentagastrin on rat parietal cells' by Brenna, Sandvik and Waldum, the authors whant to show that pentagastrin stimulates histamine release from ECL cells. Maybe this is done in two out of eight preparations, but one of these two is a parietal cell enriched fraction. Apperently only a two-fold enrichment of parietal cells was obtained, which may not be sufficiently different from non-enriched cells? The authors discuss whether the receptors are intact or not on the ECL cells.This is a very central problem to solve before it is useful to discuss the presence or absence of receptors on any cell.

The paper contains 5 figures and 3 tables. In 3-4 ~~figures the~~ results have been extracted from the tables. It is recommended by the journal that the number of figures and tables should be kept at minimum without double recording!

Three methods for staining of ECL cells are decribed in Methods but there is no indication in the Results which ones that have been used. One reference, Panula et al., is incomplete.

The authors approach an important problem but unfortunately the results are not sufficiently convincing. The text is partly unclear and poorly written, it could be considerably improved by condensing. At present the manuscript cannot be recommended for publication.

Editor E. Gjone
Scandinavian Journal of Gastroenterology
Medisinsk avdeling A
Rikshospitalet
0027 OSLO 1

02.12.91 HKW/bm

Concerning our paper:
that soon will appear in Scandinavian Journal of Gastroenterology. Our manuscript was only accepted after strong pressure and after a delay of 12 months in your Journal. I have known all the time that we have made an important work with important physiological as well as clinical implications. Accordingly I was very astonished by the reviewers comments. The reason for this letter was a recent paper in American Journal of Physiology where the same problems were studied with much of the same methodology. I think that one of your reviewers had to be one of the authors of the paper in American Journal of Physiology, since this reviewer suggested combination of high gastrin concentrations with high histamine concentration to show a separate gastrin effect on the aminopyrine uptake in isolated mucosal cells without IMX stimulation. On his advice we included this in our study too. However, this was only a minor part of the work and the relevance of these results is not obvious since the gastrin concentrations used were so high. On the other hand, our manuscript contain much more information:

We studied the effect on histamine release parallel to the effect of aminopyrine uptake, and we did do differential staining particularly with respect to the enterochromaffin-like (ECL) cell in a different fraction enriched by elutriation. It seems to me that one of the reviewers try to retard our manuscript while he on the same time was doing the work and sending the manuscript on the same problem to the American Journal of Physiology. Actually our manuscript was sent to Scandinavian Journal of Gastroenterology in August 1990 while the paper published in American Journal of Physiology was received there in December 1990. Moreover, our manuscript was initially sent to Acta Physiologica Scandinavica and refused there. I therefore enclose a copy of my letter to the Editor of this journal.

I did not know exactly what I want from the Scandinavian Journal of Gastroenterology, but I should like you to discuss this letter. It must be realized that gastric physiology has become a very hot topic where non scientific interests have more and more influence. I do, however, hope that the Editorial Board will take notice of what has happened and that you will rely more on our group than on reviewers in controversial questions. As a matter of fact the important findings that we have made in gastric physiology since 1983 and that has mainly been published in Scandinavian Journal of Gastroenterology have been shown to be correct. This is because we have the best models to study the regulation of gastric physiology, and that we are free of commersial interests.

Sincerely yours

Helge L. Waldum
Professor of Medicine
Department of Medicine
University Hospital, N-7006 Trondheim, Norway

The localization of the gastrin receptor and the disappearance of fluorescein-labelled gastrin agonists from the market

Based upon our studies on the isolated rat stomach and isolated rat oxyntic mucosal cells, it was clear that the gastrin receptor had to be localized to the ECL cell. Additionally, from a functional point of view there was no need for a gastrin receptor on the parietal cell. However, Kopin et al. cloned the gastrin receptor from oxyntic mucosal cells which had been highly enriched with parietal cells (Kopin et al. 1992).

This was taken as a proof that the gastrin receptor was localized to this cell. However, even in a highly enriched cell fraction, there are a few contaminating cells. Therefore, it is likely that in the ones that Kopin et al. used to clone the gastrin receptor, there were a few histamine-producing ECL cells. Shortly afterwards, the gastrin receptor was cloned from an ECL cell tumor by a Japanese group (Nakata et al. 1992). It is, however, problematic, as it is rare that the same signal substance is found in two consecutive types of cells in a regulatory chain.

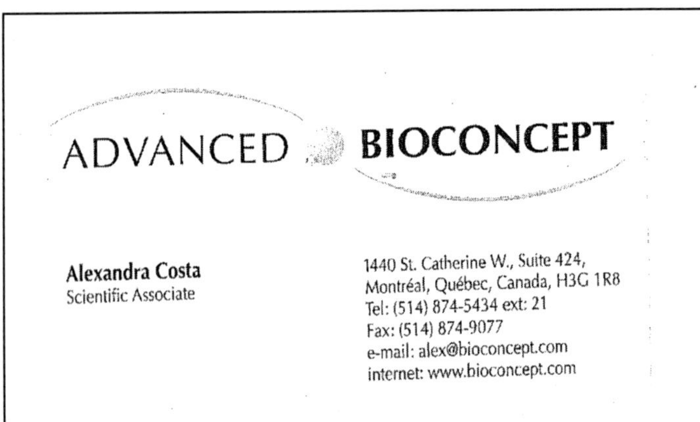

When a fluorescein-labelled gastrin analogue became available from a small new company (Advanced Bioconcept, Montreal, Quebec, Canada), we used it in a physiological concentration in the isolated rat's stomach, which we rapidly put into liquid nitrogen and examined for fluorescein and cell types using immunohistochemistry.

We found that fluorescein (gastrin) was only bound to the ECL cell, and not to the parietal cell. We first sent it to *Gut*, who refused it because the fact that the gastrin receptor was localized to the parietal cell was already known. Therefore, the journal refused the manuscript because it did not support the existing point of view, and not because they had detected any errors in the applied methods. Such an attitude will always preserve old theories, even if they are obviously incorrect. Then we sent it to the *Scandinavian Journal of Gastroenterology* where it was published (Bakke et al. 2001).

When we applied for more of the fluorescein gastrin analogue, we were told that it was not available because another pharmaceutical company had bought the entire stock. Since then, this substance has not been available and, to my knowledge, there is no report on its use by any pharmaceutical company. Therefore, it is difficult to avoid the impression that the pharmaceutical company feared that these results would appear when using this compound, and so they prevented its use.

Gut

An International Journal of Gastroenterology and Hepatology

Published by the BMJ Publishing Group

BMA HOUSE
TAVISTOCK SQUARE
LONDON WC1H 9JR

Telephone: +44 (0) 20 7383 6394/6157
Fax: +44 (0) 20 7383 6787
Email: guteditorial@bmjgroup.com
Website: www.gutjnl.com

05 December 2000

DR INGUNN BAKKE
DEPT OF PHYSIOLOGY & BIOMEDICAL ENGINEERING
FACULTY OF MEDICINE
NORWEGIAN UNIVERSITY OF SCIENCE & TECHNOLOGY
N-7489 TRONDHEIM
NORWAY

Correspondence with Gut.
Ingunn Bakke is my PhD candidate

Dear Dr Bakke

Re: GUT/2000/675 - *BIOLOGICALLY ACTIVE CCK-2 RECEPTORS ARE LOCATED ON THE ECL CELL, BUT NOT ON THE PARIETAL CELL*

Thank you for submitting this paper to *Gut,* which was discussed at the last editorial committee meeting. I am sorry to say that I am unable to accept it for publication on this occasion and return your manuscript with regret. I am enclosing the referees' comments; you may find them helpful if you wish to resubmit your manuscript to another journal.

With kind regards

Yours sincerely

Professor M J G Farthing
Editor

FRI 11:32 FAX

Comments for authors

This is a very interesting and potentially important study from authors who have contributed much to the debate regarding localization and physiology of gastrin receptors in gastric mucosa. The authors have utilized fluorescein-labelled CCK-8 to demonstrate that functional CCK-2/gastrin receptors are localized to ECL but not parietal cells. This supports the authors' previous conclusions but is in disagreement with other in situ and receptor localization studies. This discrepancy is discussed.

Major points:

1. The authors have shown that fluo-CCK-8 binding did not co-localise with parietal cells. Is it possible this is a false negative response? The authors noted that previous investigators found parietal cell but not ECL-cell gastrin receptors. Is the current result due to methodology? The authors' case would be strengthened if they simultaneously demonstrated localization of any other receptor type (histamine, muscarinic etc) to parietal cells, showing the efficacy of their methods.
2. Active CCK-1 and CCK-2 receptors are believed to be located on fundic D-cells. It would be expected that fluo-CCK-8 should bind to these; can the authors demonstrate such binding? The authors seem to have only demonstrated ECL-cell binding. If the method is not detecting D-cell binding, the authors should explain this discrepancy.
3. The authors have reviewed data on in vitro effects of gastrin on parietal cells and conclude that the actions are almost certainly indirect. Other data, they do not discuss (eg Kaise et al J Biol Chem. 1995 May 12;270(19):11155-60) suggest that gastrin does directly regulate parietal cell function. The intracellular responses and the interactions with glycine-extended gastrin are consistent with other data in other cell types (which lack a H2 receptor) and suggest a parietal cell gastrin receptor.
4. The title should specify the species under investigation.
5. Membrane (P 10, L 11)

'00 FRI 11:33 FAX

Bakke et al have performed series of experiments using immuno-histochemistry to determine the localization of CCK-2 receptors in the rat oxyntic mucosa. Commercially available fluorescein labeled CCK-8 was arterially perfused through the isolated rat stomach. It was found that Fluo-CCK-8 stimulated the release of histamine from ECL cells and was therefore biologically active. Immunohistochemical analysis using antibodies against fluorescein of the Fluo-CCK-2 compound, histidine decarboxylase and H, K-ATPase showed that CCK-2 was localized to ECL cells and not parietal cells.

The rational for undertaking these experiments is the belief that the role of histamine and gastrin in the regulation of gastric acid secretion is controversial. Thirty years ago this was the case, however with the advent of the powerful techniques of molecular biology and ion imaging at the single cell level it is now clear that a gastrin receptor is located on the parietal and its stimulation results in in the activation of a signaling cascade (Athmann et al, 2000, AJP 279:G1048-1058).

Major Criticisms:

1. Only 2 animals were used in both the experimental and control conditions. More subjects in both groups would allow the use of statistical analysis.
2. The effect of Fluo-CCK-8 on histamine release to determine biological activity of the fluorescein conjugated compound was done at only a single concentration (130pM). In the results section subtitled "histamine release" it is stated that the vascular histamine concentration was of a magnitude comparable to the histamine release induced by native CCK-8. The concentration of native CCK-8 used in this study was 520nM. Were these two different concentrations used as a comparison for the biological effects? If not, where is the reference? Additionally, in the first paragraph of the Discussion section it is stated that the biological activity of Fluo-CCK-8 was tested by IC50 analysis, this is not referenced.

Minor Criticisms:

1. It is not stated in what animal the polyclonal HDC antibody was raised or what the secondary antibody was.
2. Although a normal unstimulated rat stomach was used a negative control for the anti-fluorescein immunostaining, negative controls for the HDS and HK-ATPase immunostaining experiments were not conducted. The use of normal sera in place of the antisera or preadsorbing the antibody with antigen should be done.

NTNU
Norwegian University of Science and Technology

Faculty of Medicine
Department of Intra-Abdominal Diseases

Professor M J Farthing
Editor Gut
BMJ Publishing Group
BMA House
Tavistock Square
LONDON WC1H 9JR
UK

Telephone no.:

Dated:	Our ref.:	Your letter dated:	Your ref.:
2001-01-02	HLW/bm		

Re.: Gut/2000/675 – "Biologically active CCK-2 receptors are located on the ECL cell, but not on the parietal cell"

Dear Professor Farthing,

This is not a letter asking for reconsideration of our manuscript that was refused after more than six months evaluation in your Editorial Office. However, I have always meant that it is pertinent for scientists to comment on reviewers report when they are obviously misleading. I do know that editorial offices seldomly or never do re-evaluate manuscripts although it may be obvious that serious errors have been made by the reviewers.

I have no comments on reviewer 1 that was basically positive to our manuscript. However, it must be allowed to make comments on reviewer 2 that obviously does not have sufficient knowledge within the field. Thus he referred to a recent paper by Athmann et al. AJP 2000; 279: G1048-1058, claiming that there is a CCK-2 receptor on the parietal cell. Therefore our manuscript should not be accepted.

First, this is a very dangerous scientific attitude claiming that manuscripts should be refused due to the results. If there are different results when using different methods, the differences should be tried to be explained. Moreover, in the study by Athmann that the reviewer referred to, they only found an effect of gastrin independent of stimulation of histamine release at the concentration of 10 nM gastrin, that is an non-physiological concentration. Therefore this effect could be non-specific and mediated by another receptor, for instance CCK-1 receptor. This reviewer also seems to have completely misunderstood our manuscript, which to our knowledge is the first manuscript where a physiological approach to immunohistochemical detection of the CCK-2 receptor is applied. We used the concentration of 100 pM (0.1 nM), which is in the physiological range. Thus, reviewer 2 has completely misunderstood the results of the Athmann study, and based upon such misinterpretation he refuses our study.

Address
Regionsykehuset i Trondheim
N-7006 Trondheim
Norway

Location
Olav Kyrres g. 17
Regionsykehuset i Trondheim

Tel. +47 73 86 85 60
Fax +47 73 86 75 46
Org. no. NO 974 767 880

This reviewer also completely misunderstands histomorphometric studies. He claims that we had performed too few studies and therefore we could not do any statistical evaluation. It is correct that we did a qualitative study, but it would have been very easy to make a statistical evaluation. We could count 100 parietal cells and 100 ECL cells and see how many of these cells expressed the gastrin - CCK-2 receptor. Then we would have obtained 0 of 100 parietal cells and 100 of 100 ECL cells being positive for the CCK-2 receptor, which would be highly significant.

The other points made by this reviewer concerning our manuscript, could easily be checked and included in the manuscript.

In conclusion, reviewer 2 has not understood the study of Athmann where the effect of gastrin at the concentration of 1 nM on parietal cells could be completely inhibited by a histamine 2 receptor antagonist, that is the effect was mediated by histamine release, which is completely in agreement with our study where we used the concentration of 0.1 nM. In other words, neither we nor Athmann found any indications of any physiological CCK-2 receptor on the parietal cells. The effect on parietal cells of gastrin at the concentration of 10 nM which could not be inhibited by the histamine 2 receptor blocker, must have been mediated by another receptor. The claim for a statistical evaluation shows at best that the reviewer has not understood our study.

I am writing this letter to make you aware of these points. I do know that it will reduce our possibility to have anything published in Gut in the future, but nevertheless I do mean that reviewers should not be allowed to come up with false statements to stop manuscripts due to personal or other reasons.

Sincerely yours,

Helge L. Waldum
Professor of Medicine

Page 2 of 2
farthing. gut. biologically active cck-2. 28.12.doc

The trophic effect of gastrin on the ECL cell

There seems to be a general principle that stimulating a cell's function is also accompanied by stimulating proliferation, but only if the cell can divide. Gastrin was known to stimulate the oxyntic mucosa's function (acid secretion) and, since the fifties, it has also been suspected that it can stimulate cell growth, based upon experiences with patients suffering from a gastrin producing tumor, known as Zollinger-Ellison syndrome (Zollinger and Ellison 1955). In the sixties, experimental animal studies supported the view that gastrin had a generally positive trophic effect on oxyntic mucosa.

Eventually, in the early eighties, it was recognized that gastrin has a specific positive trophic effect on the ECL cell, because patients with atrophic gastritis and secondary hypergastrinemia (Borch, Renvall, and Liedberg 1985), as well as patients with gastrinoma (Solcia et al. 1990), developed tumors originating from this cell. At the same time as we demonstrated that gastrin stimulated acid secretion by inducing histamine release from the ECL cell (Sandvik et al. 1987), there were reports describing how rodents, that had been dosed long-term with efficient inhibitors of acid secretion, such as proton pump inhibitors (PPIs) (Havu 1986) or the histamine-2 blocker loxtidine (Poynter et al. 1986), which both lead to hypergastrinemia, developed tumors originating from the ECL cell. Also, there is apparently a close correlation between function and growth when we consider the effects of gastrin on the ECL cell.

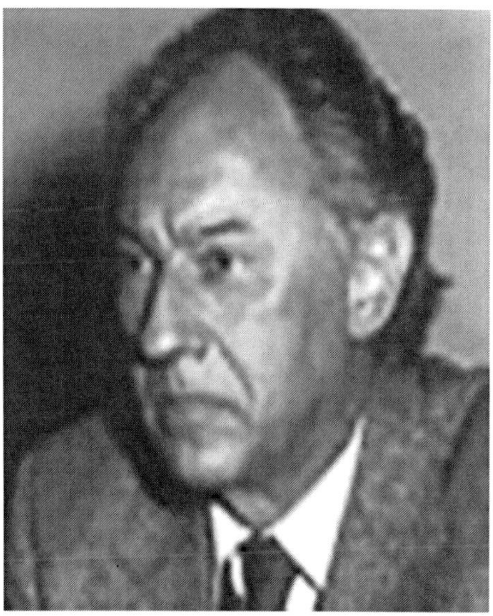

Professor Serge Bonfils
Photo: by permission of INSERM, France

I spent 1987–88 in Paris at Hôpital Bichat, which was headed by Professor Bonfils, who was the undisputed "King" of French gastroenterology, as he had supervised most of the professors within his field in France. Based upon our findings with the isolated rat stomach, as well as the descriptions of ECL cell derived tumors in patients with long-term hypergastrinemia, I pointed out that that I had begun to doubt the presence of a gastrin receptor on the parietal cell during an oral examination. Professor Bonfils turned pale, and the next day I received a handwritten 5-page letter, where he stated that he regretted taking me into the unit. This made me realize the great importance and potential of gastrin's trophic effect, and that we had to research not only its function but also its role in the development of neoplasia. During my stay in Paris, I followed a course on gastrointestinal physiology and passed four examinations (two oral and two written), which I benefitted from in my later studies.

When I returned home, I immediately sat up animal experiments to study gastrin's trophic effects. By continuously giving gastrin to rats using osmotic "minipumps" for three months, we could show that the maximal trophic effect occurred at a lower gastrin concentration than had previously been thought, and that there was a similar concentration dependency for both functional and trophic effects. The manuscript was sent to *Gastroenterology* and had practically been accepted for publication (with minor changes), when there was a change of editor. The new editor unexpectedly refused the manuscript, which was then later published in another journal (Brenna and Waldum 1992).

The proliferation of neuroendocrine cells

In a multicellular organism, there is a differentiation between the cells acquiring specific functions. In order to coordinate the cellular functions, there is a need for regulatory systems to coordinate the cells involved. The nervous system and the endocrine cells take care of this regulation. Locally, on most external surfaces, we have neuroendocrine cells, which receive information from the nerves and the blood (hormones), as well as from the surface where they are located (neuroendocrine open type cells).

Neuroendocrine cells have axon-like projections and, morphologically, they resemble neurons (Gustafsson et al. 2011), but they also have close contact with blood vessels (hormonal activity). Moreover, they share organelles, such as secretory granules containing chromogranins, and synaptic vesicles containing synaptophysin with neural and endocrine cells.

Accordingly, when Pearse formulated his theory, it was an attractive hypothesis that neuroendocrine cells embryologically originated from the neural crest (Pearse and Polak 1971). However, in chimeric studies, Le Douarin found the neural crest origin for the pituitary endocrine cells, but not the neuroendocrine cells from the gastrointestinal tract (Le Douarin and

Teillet 1973). There have been later studies which indicate that neuroendocrine cells originate from the endodermal stem cell.

It became established early on that rodent neuroendocrine cells can proliferate, such as is the case for ECL cells (Tielemans et al. 1990). Also, it was found that in humans long-term hypergastrinemia induces selective ECL cell hyperplasia and forming localized accumulation of ECL cells as carcinoids. This indirectly shows that the ECL cells can divide. In 1995, Barrett and co-workers (including Sir Nic. Wright) published an article stating that human neuroendocrine cells do not divide (Barrett et al. 1995). However, they had obviously not examined enough cells to draw this conclusion (Waldum and Brenna 1996).

It was also established that human pancreas beta-cells divide (Dor et al. 2004). This means that the digestive system's neuroendocrine cells have a feature, which distinguishes them from other cells. Taking into consideration that all cells that can divide have the potential to create neoplasia, the question of whether they proliferate or not is of great clinical significance.

The cellular origin of tumors is very important because understanding their growth regulation could tell us a lot about their pathogenesis.

The cellular origins of tumors: Time for a paradigm shift?

The currently accepted theory of tumorigenesis is that neoplasia originate from stem cells, which stops their differentiation at a certain level, and the earlier this occurs leads to a more malignant tumor.

An alternative view is that tumors may develop from all cell types that have the ability to divide, and that they become increasingly dedifferentiated over time, which makes them more malignant (Waldum et al. 2018). The tumorigenesis process may be influenced at an early stage when the origin cell's growth regulation is understood. Therefore, in gastric carcinogenesis, gastrin may be expected to be involved in tumors originating from the ECL cell, but this is not necessarily the case for tumors originating from the stem cell, whose growth may be only indirectly affected by gastrin.

Disputes about the origin cells of tumors have practical and clinical implications, and the present understanding that all tumors develop from stem cells, which I firmly believe is incorrect, continues to significantly limit progress in the prevention and treatment of neoplasia. During the last decade, the concept of cancer stem cells has evolved (Wang et al. 2015).

According to this theory, cancer stem cells are present at an early stage of a tumor's life, and they do not change much over time. If cancers develop from differentiated cells which dedifferentiate, then patients may be cured if tumors are removed before they become too malignant. The cancer stem cell hypothesis is at odds with the well-known clinical experience that most tumors do not recur when they are removed completely at an early stage before they have the ability to invade or metastasize. There is ample evidence of a transition from hyperplasia to benign and then later malignant neoplasia in neuroendocrine tumorigenesis (Qvigstad, Falkmer, et al. 1999; Calvete et al. 2015) without any sign of a stem cell.

Thesis in Paris 1993

During my one year stay in Paris, I passed my "DEA" in gastric physiology and pathophysiology. This enabled me to write my thesis. During the last oral examination, I had a quarrel with Professor Bonfils about the interaction between the three major stimulators of acid secretion (acetylcholine, gastrin, and histamine). Bonfils used the well-known general trophic effect of gastrin on the acid producing (oxyntic) mucosa (which has been known since the first description of thick oxyntic mucosa in patients with gastrinoma in the fifties) as an argument that gastrin affected the oxyntic mucosa stem cell.

When I returned to Norway, I conducted many studies related to gastric acid secretion, the trophic control of the gastric mucosa, and the role of the ECL cell and gastrin in gastric carcinogenesis. I submitted my thesis early in 1992, and the University in Paris (Paris VII) established a committee of five of the most skilled French-speaking scientists in the field: Prof. Serge Bonfils, Prof. Michel Mignon, Prof. Daniel Cattan, Prof. Miguel Lewin, who were all from Paris, and Prof. G. Willems from Brussels.

However, the initial version was not accepted. I later heard that this was because Willems could not accept that I implicated gastrin in gastric tumorigenesis. I was, however, allowed to revise the thesis and resubmit it within one year. I then modified it slightly and it was found worthy of being defended in public, which took place in December 1993. But, even on this occasion, there was some external interference, as I heard that the producer of PPI, Astra, wanted to send a Swede to oppose it from the auditorium. This was not welcomed by my bosses in Paris and so no one turned up.

In retrospect, I regret this, as I would have had no problems defending myself scientifically and it is likely that my French would have been much better than the Swedish expert's. Anyway, the dissertation went well and it was a friendly atmosphere. Looking back, my year in Paris was of great importance for my later career and research, and I am grateful for my French connections.

The role of the ECL cell in gastric carcinogenesis

As discussed briefly above, neuroendocrine cells, including the histamine producing ECL cell, can divide and they may lead to tumors. Moreover, long-term hypergastrinemia in humans, whether due to reduced gastric acid secretion secondary to atrophic gastritis or caused by a gastrin-producing tumor accompanied by increased acid secretion, has been known to induce benign ECL cell tumors (ECL cell carcinoids) since the early eighties.

Nevertheless, Italian pathologists claim that gastrin alone could not induce tumors and that gastritis has an important role in tumor pathogenesis in patients with atrophic gastritis and anacidity. They claim that ECL-omas in patients with gastrinomas only occur if there is a genetic defect in the neuroendocrine cells, MEN I, which makes the sufferer prone to developing neuroendocrine tumors (Bordi et al. 1995). However, patients with gastrinoma without MEN I can also develop ECL cell dysplasia (Peghini et al. 2002) and ECL-omas with long-term hypergastrinemia (Feurle 1994) (Cadiot et al. 1995). Patients with gastrinoma without MEN I may be cured by an operation, or they may die earlier because their tumors are more malignant than those in MEN I patients with multiple, but often rather benign, gastrinomas. Therefore, the period of hypergastrinemia may be longer in gastrinoma patients with MEN I compared with those with sporadic gastrinoma.

Rindi and colleagues' classification of ECL cell carcinoids divides them into type 1, which occurs in patients with hypergastrinemia secondary to atrophic gastritis; type 2, which is due to hypergastrinemia in gastrinoma patients with MEN I; and type 3, which occurs in patients without hypergastrinemia (Rindi et al. 1993). This is not logical, and it should be replaced by two types of classification: ECL cell carcinoids developed in patients with long-term hypergastrinemia independent of cause, and type 2, which occurs in patients without hypergastrinemia.

In the middle of the eighties, when Astra reported the occurrence of tumors in the oxyntic mucosa of rats that had been dosed long-term with the first proton pump inhibitor (PPI), omeprazole (Havu 1986), all clinical studies using this substance were stopped. At the same time, Glaxo in England

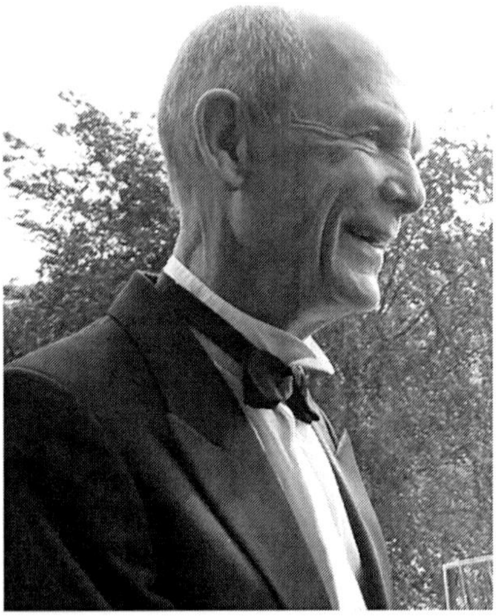
Sture Falkmer Photo: private

reported similar tumors in rodents dosed with the insurmountable histamine-2 antagonist loxtidine (Poynter et al. 1986), and it was realized that these tumors had developed due to profound acid inhibition. The tumors were initially classified as carcinomas by Glaxo, but the pathologist Nilo Havo (who was trained by neuroendocrinology expert, Sture Falkmer, who I collaborated with during his stay in Trondheim) classified them as ECL cell derived. The rodent tumors were then regarded as ECL cell carcinoids, which is a rare and rather benign human tumor.

Astra continued developing omeprazole, while Glaxo stopped working with loxtidine. During meetings with clinicians and pathologists, Astra succeeded in convincing them that rodent tumors had no relevance for humans. Nevertheless, this was the first time that a compound was accepted for clinical use after having induced tumors in its target organ in any animal (K. Wormsley, Dundee). In a way, an old medical taboo had been broken. Initially, omeprazole was accepted for the use in patients with gastrinoma or very severe peptic ulcer disease, but gradually PPIs have been used in increasing numbers of patients, often only suffering from discomfort in the epigastric area. Therefore, currently PPIs are used by a large proportion of the population.

However, from previous work we knew that the distinction between neuroendocrine carcinomas and adenocarcinomas may be difficult to prove not only due to the classification of rodent tumors following long-term dosing with efficient inhibitors of acid secretion (Poynter et al. 1986; Poynter et al. 1985), but also due to the reclassification of tumors that occur spontaneously in African Mastomys (Soga, Tazawa, and Ito 1969). Moreover, Azzopardi and Pollock (Azzopardi and Pollock 1963), as well as other pathologists, had previously described the reclassification of human adenocarcinomas to neuroendocrine carcinomas. Therefore, we felt that there was reason to examine gastric carcinomas for ECL differentiation. In 1989, with the help of the bioengineer, Reidun Meczei, we started to re-examine ten diffuse-type gastric carcinomas and ten intestinal type, which had previously been classified according to Laurén (Lauren 1965).

One of these tumors was found in a young woman (about 30 years old) who had suffered from meal-induced erythema during the previous year. The skin problem was thought to be hives. Immunohistochemical examinations of this patient's gastric cancer, which was a diffuse type, showed that most of the cancer cells were positive for neuroendocrine markers, including markers specific to ECL cells. Therefore, this tumor was definitely a highly malignant ECL cell derived cancer. In a proportion of the other diffuse-type carcinomas, there were also some cancer cells that showed neuroendocrine markers. This means that the ECL cell did not seem to be unimportant when considering human gastric carcinogenesis. A manuscript based on these findings was sent to scientific journals, but it was met with hostility. Finally, I sent it to the *European Journal of Gastroenterology and Hepatology* and it initially received very negative reports.

I recognized the reviewers, and as I knew they had close connections to Astra, I wrote a letter to the Editor, stating that it was a pity that scientists with allegiances to the pharmaceutical industry could block important findings which had great implications for clinical drug use without scientific arguments. The Editor (Misiewicz) accepted the manuscript following this letter (Waldum, Haugen, et al. 1991). However, the manuscript was met with silence and nobody mentioned it, although it was very relevant to the use of PPIs.

A meeting in Trondheim: "Histamine and the stomach"

At that time, I had a good relationship with Glaxo, who produced the histamine-2 blocker, ranitidine, which was the most sold drug for a number of years until omeprazole took its place. From a scientific point of view, I favored ranitidine because it does not have such a profound inhibitory effect on gastric acid secretion. With financial support from Glaxo, in 1990 I managed to arrange an international meeting in Trondheim related to histamine and the ECL cell entitled, "Histamine and the stomach" (*Histamine and the Stomach* 1991).

I succeeded gathering all the leading persons within the field at this meeting, and, in many ways, the book that was published from it is still up-to-date (*Histamine and the Stomach* 1991). Scientists with close relations to Astra attended the meeting, and one of them said when leaving that "This has been a good meeting, and you are good at physiology, but stay out of pathology".

That, of course, made me become even more interested in pathology, which has been one of my main research areas for the last 25 years.

Long before biobanks became popular, we started to collect material from gastric tumors at the surgical theatre. We prepared and collected them in a way that would allow us to study them not only using histochemical and immunohistochemical methods, but also with electron microscopy and gene expression analysis. Moreover, we collected blood from the same patients in a fasting state for future analysis. When we had collected tissue and blood from 50 patients, we published our first study based on this material (Waldum et al. 1998). We confirmed that there was neuroendocrine and, more specifically, ECL differentiation in diffuse-type gastric carcinomas. Professor Julia Pollack, who had the Chair after Professor Pearse (who formulated the neural crest theory for the embryological origin of neuroendocrine cells), participated in this publication. Julia Pollack was an authority within neuroendocrinology, and she had published more than one thousand papers.

We then started to use the tyramide signal amplification method and we were able to show that a greater part of human gastric carcinomas showed neuroendocrine/ECL cell differentiation (Qvigstad et al. 2000). We were also able to demonstrate that virtually all tumors occurring in patients with marked hypergastrinemia (atrophic gastritis leading to pernicious anemia) originated from an ECL cell (Qvigstad et al. 2002). Similarly, virtually all gastric carcinomas from the subgroup of diffuse gastric carcinomas, where the tumor cells resemble a signet-ring, were shown to express neuroendocrine markers (Bakkelund et al. 2006). Likewise, even though we used immunohistochemistry and in situ hybridization, we could not detect any trace of mucin expression in the signet ring cancer cells, which further supports the view that these cancers are not adenocarcinomas, but are instead neuroendocrine carcinomas (Sordal et al. 2014).

Therefore, the ECL cell is important in human gastric carcinogenesis, and the premise for taking PPIs into clinical use is not correct. Surprisingly few people have been interested in these aspects and most of our manuscripts on this subject have been met with hostility or neglected. As I see it, the resistance to our studies and findings is due to the following factors:

1. The influence of the pharmaceutical industry on medical science. During a meeting in the Swedish city of Södertälje, which had been arranged by Astra in the late eighties, many influential clinicians and pathologists came to the consensus that the ECL cell was of minor importance to human gastric

carcinogenesis. For some reason or other, those attending this meeting have stuck to this conclusion.

2. Pathologists stick to the dogma that PAS positivity is specific for mucin, and that a PAS positive cell implies an exocrine origin.

3. Although there is ample evidence that chronic hormonal overstimulation may induce tumors from target cells, presently most scientists still believe that hormones alone do not cause malignant tumors, but only promote the growth of cells otherwise changed by mutation. In other words, most scientists have not taken into consideration that every mitosis implies a risk of mutation, which means that mitogens are also mutagens.

4. The dogma that all malignant tumors originate from stem cells. Therefore, we are not only fighting strong economic interests, but also old paradigms.

FEB-13-'90 TUE 10:04 ID:AM CANCER SOC A2X??I TEL NO: #118 P01

Cancer

A Journal of the American Cancer Society, Inc.

Editor: Jonathan E. Rhoads, M.D., D.Sc.(Med)
Hospital of the University of Pennsylvania
3400 Spruce Street
Philadelphia, Pennsylvania 19104

Phone: 215-662-2017
FAX: 215-349-5849

February 14, 1990

Dr. H. L. Waldum
Department of Medicine
University Hospital of Trondheim
N-7006 Trondheim
Norway

Dear Dr. Waldum:

Your manuscript, "Are diffuse gastric carcinomas neuro-endocrine tumours (ECL-OMAS)?", has been returned by our reviewers, and I am sorry to tell you that they have not recommended that it be accepted for publication in CANCER.

We are, therefore, returning your paper to you so that you may submit it elsewhere if you should care to do so. Thank you for submitting your paper to us. We appreciate your interest in CANCER, and regret that we are unable to be of service to you in this instance.

Sincerely yours,

Jonathan E. Rhoads, MD

NOV-29-'89 WED 10:11 ID:AM CANCER SOC A2X/?F TEL NO: #029 P01

DEAR DR. WALDUM: THE COMMENTS BELOW REPRESENT THE CRITIQUES OF BOTH REVIEWERS. WE HOPE THAT THEY ARE OF SOME HELP TO YOU IN SUBMITTING YOUR WORK ELSEWHERE.

47 7 597977

nov 89

Comments: In 1969 Toker (Cancer: 24: 256-260, 1989) pointed out that the 'anaplastic' areas of colonic carcinomas actually represented a carcinoidal component. He indicated, too, that it was probab ly universally true that most tumours were composites - containing both exocrine and endocrine elements.

The present study, utilizing unreliable and complicated methodology, adds nothing to this earlier work, which depended on the accurate and perceptive application of a simple and dependable modality - the H&E section.

With regard to hypoacidity and gastric carcinoma, it may be pointed out

OVER

out that a relationship between the two has been recognized for decades. It is well known that gastric carcinomas may occur in patients who have had subtotal gastrectomies, and in patients with pernicious anaemia. What the authors did not do, and what may well have been a valuable contribution, was to investigate the backgrounds of the cancer patients in their own study, in order to establish whether these patients had been subjected to prolonged antacid therapy.

Suggested Recommendations:

JCb 90

____ Accept as submitted
____ Accept with minor revisions
____ Accept with major revisions
____ Reject but recommend resubmission following revision or inclusion of more data
_X_ Reject
____ Recommend that the paper be published as a lead article
____ Recommend that the paper be published as soon as possible
____ Submit it to another (more appropriate) journal

Comments: This is a rather simple study on diffuse gastric carcinoma that asks whether they are neuroendocrine (NE) tumors (ECL-omas). In my view, and in the context of 1990, this study is fundamentally flawed for it does not seriously consider the issue of carcinomas of mixed exocrine-NE phenotypes; the literature-light microscopy, electron microscopy and immunocytochemistry-on this subject is abundant and readily available. This "bypassing" is even more surprising as this very study shows that all diffuse gastric carcinomas studied had AB/PAS positive cells!

UNIVERSITETET I TRONDHEIM
DET MEDISINSKE FAKULTET
MEDISINSK AVDELING
GASTROENTEROLOGISK SEKSJON

Vår dato 15.02.90 – referanse HLW/bm
Deres dato – referanse

The Editor Jonathan E. Rhoads
Hospital of the University of Pennsylvania
3400 Spruce Street
Philadelphia
Pennsylvania 19104
USA

Thank you for your work with my manuscript: "Are diffuse gastric carcinomas neuroendocrine tumours (ECL-omas)?".

I hope you noticed that the 2 first reviewers found the method too complex while the last one described the study rather simple. It is strange that the latter did not realize that my study could mean that the diffuse gastric carcinomas actually were "pure" neuroendocrine tumours. It should also be mentioned that I gave an explanation for the PAS-positivity of the tumour cells. We stated that PAS-positivity does not say that there is mucous-production in the cell, since PAS stains glycoproteins. Time will show who was right.

Sincerely yours

Helge L. Waldum
Professor of Medicine
Department of Medicine
University Hospital
N-7006 Trondheim
NORWAY

POSTADRESSE
REGIONSYKEHUSET I TRONDHEIM
N-7000 TRONDHEIM

TELEFON
(07) 59 74 63
INT. TLF.NR.
-47 7 59 74 63

THE UNIVERSITY OF TRONDHEIM
FACULTY OF MEDICINE
DEPARTMENT OF MEDICINE
SECTION OF GASTROENTEROLOGY
TRONDHEIM REGIONAL HOSPITAL
N-7000 TRONDHEIM, NORWAY

The role of gastric juice in the defense against prion infections

The main function of gastric juice is to kill swallowed microorganisms. It is uniquely suited to this task because it is a strong acid with active enzymes.

Prions are infectious proteins which are very resistant to destruction (Mould, Dawson, and Smith 1965). Therefore, they can withstand quite strong heat and very strong acid. Gastric juice is believed to not affect the susceptibility to prion diseases due to the latter property. Prion diseases are mainly chronic, progressive, neural diseases with a long latency, such as Creutzfeldt-Jacob disease and kuru, but prions could also be involved in the pathogenesis of prevalent and debilitating diseases, such as Alzheimer's disease and Parkinson's disease (Prusiner 2012).

There is every reason to believe that prion diseases are acquired via the oral route. Due to the development of variant Creutzfeldt-Jacob disease in some individuals after consuming contaminated meat (Will et al. 1996), we wanted to explore whether native gastric juice, which also contains active enzymes, could reduce susceptibility to prion infection in contrast to in vitro studies with acid alone. In two consecutive studies in mice, we found evidence for a protective role of gastric juice with respect to prion infection (Martinsen et al. 2002; Martinsen et al. 2011). Again, these studies were not considered positively and have been neglected.

Rebound acid hypersecretion

Quickly after PPIs entered into clinical use, many clinicians found that their patients had difficulties in stopping the treatment, when it had continued for some time. Some suspected that the treatment could induce rebound acid hypersecretion, which increased acid secretion after the treatment period compared to before starting treatment. However, the initial studies did not show any evidence of a rebound effect after the use of PPIs (Prewett et al. 1991), although a short-lived rebound effect was detected following the use of less efficient histamine-2 blockers (Fullarton et al. 1989).

Based on our studies with the isolated rat stomach, we knew that the maximum histamine stimulated acid secretion exceeded that of gastrin (Kleveland, Waldum, and Larsson 1987), and that gastrin stimulated acid secretion by inducing histamine release from the ECL cell. Moreover, it was known that gastrin had a positive trophic effect on the ECL cell.

We started a study on rats, where we gave a high dose of omeprazole for three months, then we stopped the dosing for three days, and removed their stomachs for examination in the isolated rat stomach model. We found that gastrin increased the ECL density and histamine release, while acid secretion, surprisingly, was not increased (Waldum, Lehy, et al. 1991). Shortly afterwards, we realized that the effect of the PPI on acid secretion persisted for a longer than three days. In addition, we treated patients with reflux esophagitis for three months with a normal dose of omeprazole and examined acid secretion before beginning and two weeks after the cessation of treatment. We could then detect a marked increase in acid secretion compared to the pre-treatment value: i.e., rebound acid hypersecretion (Waldum, Arnestad, et al. 1996).

In fact, some years before Håkan Larsson had described rebound acid hypersecretion after the administration of omeprazole to rats (Larsson et al. 1988), but Astra did not focus on this phenomenon. Since it is known that increased gastric acid secretion worsens gastro-esophageal reflux, I never doubted that the rebound might have negative effects on patients. However, I felt it would be unfortunate to do a study on humans to show it, particularly when it requires giving healthy volunteers PPIs over a long period. However, a Danish group did this, and recorded symptoms before, during, and after the dosing period. Not unexpectedly, many of the students developed dyspeptic symptoms some days after stopping the drug (Reimer et al. 2009).

Accordingly, there is no doubt that PPI induced rebound acid hypersecretion has clinical consequences, and that the problems when stopping PPI treatment (Bjornsson et al. 2006) are likely to be related to this phenomenon. It should also be added that there have been discussions over whether to initiate treatment with the most efficient inhibitors of acid secretion, PPIs, or the less efficient histamine-2 blockers. However, we showed that histamine-2 blockers lost potency after a period with PPIs, due to the increased concentrations of histamine in gastric mucosa (Qvigstad et al. 1998). Therefore, the correct way would be to start with histamine-2 blockers in mild to moderate reflux disease.

Helicobacter pylori

I was slow to accept Helicobacter pylori (Hp) as the cause of peptic ulcer disease because I could not understand how a bacterial infection could induce a localized disease which tended to recur at the same location. In fact, for some years, I had firmly believed that the viral infection in neural ganglia, which was parallel to herpes virus infections at other locations, was the cause of peptic ulcer disease (Waldum, Bjorvatn, and Burhol 1981). First, after the description of increased gastric acidity secondary to antral Hp infection with hypergastrinemia (Levi et al. 1989), I realized that in reality Hp was the main cause of peptic ulcer disease as well as chronic gastritis. Since gastric cancer was known to occur almost exclusively in stomachs with gastritis (Morson 1955), it was no surprise that Hp gastritis was also recognized as a major gastric carcinogen (Parsonnet et al. 1991). Hp produces urease which leads to NH_3 formation by splitting urea (Marshall et al. 1990); this in turn elevates the pH in the antral mucosa and accordingly reduces the inhibition of gastrin release. This means that gastric acid secretion is increased, which is a hallmark of duodenal ulcer disease (Wormsley and Grossman 1965) and indicates a predisposition to such ulcers. Gastric ulcers, on the other hand, are due to the reduced mucosal defense mechanisms caused by gastritis, which leads to ulcerations (Byrd et al. 2000). Accordingly, the pathogenesis of Hp in gastritis, as well as gastric and duodenal ulcers, is clearly understood. However, the mechanism for the carcinogenic effect of Hp gastritis is not yet understood despite 30-years' worth of intensive research. However, Uemura et al. made the important discovery that Hp gastritis predisposed a patient to gastric cancer only after having induced oxyntic atrophy (Uemura et al. 2001). This suggested that the carcinogenic effect was related to reduced gastric acidity, which limits the destruction of swallowed microorganisms and induces secondary hypergastrinemia. If microbes were the carcinogenic factor, one would then expect that the increased cancer risk would be uniform throughout the stomach, which is not the case. In patients with autoimmune gastritis, carcinomas occur almost exclusively in the oxyntic mucosa rather than the antral mucosa (Zamcheck et al. 1955). In addition, Hp infection has less of a carcinogenic effect on the cardiac mucosa (Parsonnet et al. 1991). Therefore, hypergastrinemia provoked by Hp induced oxyntic atrophy, seems to be the most plausible mechanism as we suggested in 1994(Waldum, Sandvik, and Brenna 1993) and then elaborated on at a later date (Waldum et al. 2015). However, incriminating gastrin in gastric tumourigenesis/carcinogenesis, whether due to oxyntic atrophic gastritis from autoimmunity, Helicobacter pylori, or gastrinoma, has been unpopular just like the role of the ECL cell in human gastric carcinoids and carcinomas. This is peculiar since this was not the case before the introduction of PPIs into clinical medicine (Azzopardi and Pollock 1963; Wilander 1980).

Conclusion

Throughout the years, we have been met with hostility and we have been neglected. I find this peculiar because the disagreements represent science and should not be taken personally. However, because virtually no one else has worked with these problems, it has allowed us to explore the whole area. Our ideas have often proved to be correct due to our physiological knowledge. Clinical medicine should not only be based on human studies, but also on animal studies and physiological knowledge.

References

Azzopardi, J. G., and D. J. Pollock. 1963. "ARGENTAFFIN AND ARGYROPHIL CELLS IN GASTRIC CARCINOMA." *J Pathol Bacteriol* 86: 443-51.

Bakke, I., G. Qvigstad, A. K. Sandvik, and H. L. Waldum. 2001. "The CCK-2 receptor is located on the ECL cell, but not on the parietal cell." *Scand J Gastroenterol* 36 (11): 1128-33.

Bakkelund, K., R. Fossmark, I. Nordrum, and H. Waldum. 2006. "Signet ring cells in gastric carcinomas are derived from neuroendocrine cells." *J Histochem Cytochem* 54 (6): 615-21. https://doi.org/10.1369/jhc.5A6806.2005.

Barrett, P., R. C. Hobbs, P. J. Coates, R. A. Risdon, N. A. Wright, and P. A. Hall. 1995. "Endocrine cells of the human gastrointestinal tract have no proliferative capacity." *Histochem J* 27 (6): 482-6.

Berglindh, T., H. F. Helander, and K. J. Obrink. 1976. "Effects of secretagogues on oxygen consumption, aminopyrine accumulation and morphology in isolated gastric glands." *Acta Physiol Scand* 97 (4): 401-14. https://doi.org/10.1111/j.1748-1716.1976.tb10281.x.

Bjornsson, E., H. Abrahamsson, M. Simren, N. Mattsson, C. Jensen, P. Agerforz, and A. Kilander. 2006. "Discontinuation of proton pump inhibitors in patients on long-term therapy: a double-blind, placebo-controlled trial." *Aliment Pharmacol Ther* 24 (6): 945-54. https://doi.org/10.1111/j.1365-2036.2006.03084.x.

Borch, K., H. Renvall, and G. Liedberg. 1985. "Gastric endocrine cell hyperplasia and carcinoid tumors in pernicious anemia." *Gastroenterology* 88 (3): 638-48.

Bordi, C., T. D'Adda, C. Azzoni, F. P. Pilato, and P. Caruana. 1995. "Hypergastrinemia and gastric enterochromaffin-like cells." *Am J Surg Pathol* 19 Suppl 1: S8-19.

Brenna, E., and H. L. Waldum. 1991. "Studies of isolated parietal and enterochromaffin-like cells from the rat." *Scand J Gastroenterol* 26 (12): 1295-306.

—. 1992. "Trophic effect of gastrin on the enterochromaffin like cells of the rat stomach: establishment of a dose response relationship." *Gut* 33 (10): 1303-6.

Byrd, J. C., C. K. Yunker, Q. S. Xu, L. R. Sternberg, and R. S. Bresalier. 2000. "Inhibition of gastric mucin synthesis by Helicobacter pylori." *Gastroenterology* 118 (6): 1072-9. https://doi.org/10.1016/s0016-5085(00)70360-x.

Cadiot, G., C. Vissuzaine, F. Potet, and M. Mignon. 1995. "Fundic argyrophil carcinoid tumor in a patient with sporadic-type Zollinger-Ellison syndrome." *Dig Dis Sci* 40 (6): 1275-8. https://doi.org/10.1007/bf02065537.

Calvete, O., J. Reyes, S. Zuniga, B. Paumard-Hernandez, V. Fernandez, L. Bujanda, M. S. Rodriguez-Pinilla, J. Palacios, D. Heine-Suner, S. Banka, W. G. Newman, M. Canamero, D. M. Pritchard, and J. Benitez. 2015. "Exome sequencing identifies ATP4A gene as responsible of an atypical familial type I gastric neuroendocrine tumour." *Hum Mol Genet* 24 (10): 2914-22. https://doi.org/10.1093/hmg/ddv054.

Dor, Y., J. Brown, O. I. Martinez, and D. A. Melton. 2004. "Adult pancreatic beta-cells are formed by self-duplication rather than stem-cell differentiation." *Nature* 429 (6987): 41-6. https://doi.org/10.1038/nature02520.

Durant, G. J., W. A. Duncan, C. R. Ganellin, M. E. Parsons, R. C. Blakemore, and A. C. Rasmussen. 1978. "Impromidine (SK&F 92676) is a very potent and specific agonist for histamine H2 receptors." *Nature* 276 (5686): 403-5. https://doi.org/10.1038/276403a0.

Feurle, G. E. 1994. "Argyrophil cell hyperplasia and a carcinoid tumour in the stomach of a patient with sporadic Zollinger-Ellison syndrome." *Gut* 35 (2): 275-7. https://doi.org/10.1136/gut.35.2.275.

Fullarton, G. M., G. McLauchlan, A. Macdonald, G. P. Crean, and K. E. McColl. 1989. "Rebound nocturnal hypersecretion after four weeks treatment with an H2 receptor antagonist." *Gut* 30 (4): 449-54. https://doi.org/10.1136/gut.30.4.449.

Gustafsson, B. I., I. Bakke, O. Hauso, M. Kidd, I. M. Modlin, R. Fossmark, E. Brenna, and H. L. Waldum. 2011. "Parietal cell activation by arborization of ECL cell cytoplasmic projections is likely the mechanism for histamine induced secretion of hydrochloric acid." *Scand J Gastroenterol* 46 (5): 531-7. https://doi.org/10.3109/00365521.2011.558113.

Havu, N. 1986. "Enterochromaffin-like cell carcinoids of gastric mucosa in rats after life-long inhibition of gastric secretion." *Digestion* 35 Suppl 1: 42-55. https://doi.org/10.1159/000199381.

Histamine and the Stomach. 1991. Vol. Volume 26, Supplement 180.*Scandinavian Journal of Gastroenterology*, edited by H. L. Waldum and H. Petersen. Oslo: Universitetsforlaget.

Kay, A. W. 1953. "Effect of large doses of histamine on gastric secretion of HCI; an augmented histamine test." *Br Med J* 2 (4827): 77-80. https://doi.org/10.1136/bmj.2.4827.77.

Kleveland, P. M., S. E. Haugen, and H. L. Waldum. 1986. "Effect of pentagastrin on gastric acid secretion in the totally isolated vascularly perfused rat stomach stimulated with the phosphodiesterase inhibitor isobutyl methylxanthine." *Scand J Gastroenterol* 21 (5): 577-84. https://doi.org/10.3109/00365528609003103.

Kleveland, P. M., H. L. Waldum, and H. Larsson. 1987. "Gastric acid secretion in the totally isolated, vascularly perfused rat stomach. A selective muscarinic-1 agent does, whereas gastrin does not, augment maximal histamine-stimulated acid secretion." *Scand J Gastroenterol* 22 (6): 705-13. https://doi.org/10.3109/00365528709011147.

Kopin, A. S., Y. M. Lee, E. W. McBride, L. J. Miller, M. Lu, H. Y. Lin, L. F. Kolakowski, Jr., and M. Beinborn. 1992. "Expression cloning and characterization of the canine parietal cell gastrin receptor." *Proc Natl Acad Sci U S A* 89 (8): 3605-9.

Larsson, H., E. Carlsson, B. Ryberg, J. Fryklund, and B. Wallmark. 1988. "Rat parietal cell function after prolonged inhibition of gastric acid secretion." *Am J Physiol* 254 (1 Pt 1): G33-9. https://doi.org/10.1152/ajpgi.1988.254.1.G33.

Lauren, P. 1965. "The two histological main types of gastric carcinoma: Diffuse and so-called intestinal-type carcinoma. An attemt at a histo-clinical classification." *Acta Pathol Microbiol Scand* 64: 31-49.

Le Douarin, N. M., and M. A. Teillet. 1973. "The migration of neural crest cells to the wall of the digestive tract in avian embryo." *J Embryol Exp Morphol* 30 (1): 31-48.

Levi, S., K. Beardshall, G. Haddad, R. Playford, P. Ghosh, and J. Calam. 1989. "Campylobacter pylori and duodenal ulcers: the gastrin link." *Lancet* 1 (8648): 1167-8. https://doi.org/10.1016/s0140-6736(89)92752-9.

Lorenz, W., K. Thon, H. Stoltzing, E. Neugebauer, R. Lindlar, J. Sattler, and D. Weber. 1991. "Histamine and the stomach: chemical histamine assays." *Scand J Gastroenterol Suppl* 180: 9-25. https://doi.org/10.3109/00365529109093173.

Marshall, B. J., L. J. Barrett, C. Prakash, R. W. McCallum, and R. L. Guerrant. 1990. "Urea protects Helicobacter (Campylobacter) pylori from the bactericidal effect of acid." *Gastroenterology* 99 (3): 697-702. https://doi.org/10.1016/0016-5085(90)90957-3.

Martinsen, T. C., S. L. Benestad, T. Moldal, and H. L. Waldum. 2011. "Inhibitors of gastric acid secretion increase the risk of prion infection in mice." *Scand J Gastroenterol* 46 (12): 1418-22. https://doi.org/10.3109/00365521.2011.619277.

Martinsen, T. C., D. M. Taylor, R. Johnsen, and H. L. Waldum. 2002. "Gastric acidity protects mice against prion infection?" *Scand J Gastroenterol* 37 (5): 497-500. https://doi.org/10.1080/00365520252903017.

Morel, A. M., and M. A. Delaage. 1988. "Immunoanalysis of histamine through a novel chemical derivatization." *J Allergy Clin Immunol* 82 (4): 646-54. https://doi.org/10.1016/0091-6749(88)90978-5.

Morson, B. C. 1955. "Intestinal metaplasia of the gastric mucosa." *Br J Cancer* 9 (3): 365-76. https://doi.org/10.1038/bjc.1955.35.

Mould, D. L., A. M. Dawson, and W. Smith. 1965. "SCRAPIE IN MICE. THE STABILITY OF THE AGENT TO VARIOUS SUSPENDING MEDIA, PH AND SOLVENT EXTRACTION." *Res Vet Sci* 6: 151-4.

Nakata, H., T. Matsui, M. Ito, T. Taniguchi, Y. Naribayashi, N. Arima, A. Nakamura, Y. Kinoshita, K. Chihara, S. Hosoda, and et al. 1992. "Cloning and characterization of gastrin receptor from ECL carcinoid tumor of Mastomys natalensis." *Biochem Biophys Res Commun* 187 (2): 1151-7.

Parsonnet, J., G. D. Friedman, D. P. Vandersteen, Y. Chang, J. H. Vogelman, N. Orentreich, and R. K. Sibley. 1991. "Helicobacter pylori infection and the risk of gastric carcinoma." *N Engl J Med* 325 (16): 1127-31. https://doi.org/10.1056/nejm199110173251603.

Pearse, A. G., and J. M. Polak. 1971. "Neural crest origin of the endocrine polypeptide (APUD) cells of the gastrointestinal tract and pancreas." *Gut* 12 (10): 783-8. https://doi.org/10.1136/gut.12.10.783.

Peghini, P. L., B. Annibale, C. Azzoni, M. Milione, V. D. Corleto, F. Gibril, D. J. Venzon, G. Delle Fave, C. Bordi, and R. T. Jensen. 2002. "Effect of chronic hypergastrinemia on human enterochromaffin-like cells: insights from patients with sporadic gastrinomas." *Gastroenterology* 123 (1): 68-85. https://doi.org/10.1053/gast.2002.34231.

Poynter, D., C. R. Pick, R. A. Harcourt, S. A. Selway, G. Ainge, I. W. Harman, N. W. Spurling, P. A. Fluck, and J. L. Cook. 1985. "Association of long lasting unsurmountable histamine H2 blockade and gastric carcinoid tumours in the rat." *Gut* 26 (12): 1284-95.

Poynter, D., S. A. Selway, S. A. Papworth, and S. R. Riches. 1986. "Changes in the gastric mucosa of the mouse associated with long lasting unsurmountable histamine H2 blockade." *Gut* 27 (11): 1338-46. https://doi.org/10.1136/gut.27.11.1338.

Prewett, E. J., M. Hudson, C. U. Nwokolo, A. M. Sawyerr, and R. E. Pounder. 1991. "Nocturnal intragastric acidity during and after a period of dosing with either ranitidine or omeprazole." *Gastroenterology* 100 (4): 873-7. https://doi.org/10.1016/0016-5085(91)90258-m.

Prinz, C., M. Kajimura, D. R. Scott, F. Mercier, H. F. Helander, and G. Sachs. 1993. "Histamine secretion from rat enterochromaffinlike cells." *Gastroenterology* 105 (2): 449-61.

Prusiner, S. B. 2012. "Cell biology. A unifying role for prions in neurodegenerative diseases." *Science* 336 (6088): 1511-3. https://doi.org/10.1126/science.1222951.

Qvigstad, G., J. S. Arnestad, E. Brenna, and H. L. Waldum. 1998. "Treatment with proton pump inhibitors induces tolerance to histamine-2 receptor antagonists in Helicobacter pylori-negative patients." *Scand J Gastroenterol* 33 (12): 1244-8. https://doi.org/10.1080/00365529850172313.

Qvigstad, G., M. Bjorgaas, I. Eide, A. K. Sandvik, and H. L. Waldum. 1999. "Vagal stimulation augments maximal (penta) gastrin-stimulated acid secretion in humans." *Acta Physiol Scand* 165 (3): 277-81. https://doi.org/10.1046/j.1365-201x.1999.00514.x.

Qvigstad, G., S. Falkmer, B. Westre, and H. L. Waldum. 1999. "Clinical and histopathological tumour progression in ECL cell carcinoids ("ECLomas")." *Apmis* 107 (12): 1085-92.

Qvigstad, G., T. Qvigstad, B. Westre, A. K. Sandvik, E. Brenna, and H. L. Waldum. 2002. "Neuroendocrine differentiation in gastric adenocarcinomas associated with severe hypergastrinemia and/or pernicious anemia." *Apmis* 110 (2): 132-9. https://doi.org/10.1034/j.1600-0463.2002.100302.x.

Qvigstad, G., A. K. Sandvik, E. Brenna, S. Aase, and H. L. Waldum. 2000. "Detection of chromogranin A in human gastric adenocarcinomas using a sensitive immunohistochemical technique." *Histochem J* 32 (9): 551-6.

Reimer, C., B. Sondergaard, L. Hilsted, and P. Bytzer. 2009. "Proton-pump inhibitor therapy induces acid-related symptoms in healthy volunteers after withdrawal of therapy." *Gastroenterology* 137 (1): 80-7, 87.e1. https://doi.org/10.1053/j.gastro.2009.03.058.

Rindi, G., O. Luinetti, M. Cornaggia, C. Capella, and E. Solcia. 1993. "Three subtypes of gastric argyrophil carcinoid and the gastric neuroendocrine carcinoma: a clinicopathologic study." *Gastroenterology* 104 (4): 994-1006. https://doi.org/10.1016/0016-5085(93)90266-f.

Sandvik, A. K., H. L. Waldum, P. M. Kleveland, and B. Schulze Sognen. 1987. "Gastrin produces an immediate and dose-dependent histamine release preceding acid secretion in the totally isolated, vascularly perfused rat stomach." *Scand J Gastroenterol* 22 (7): 803-8. https://doi.org/10.3109/00365528708991918.

Short, G. M., M. M. Wolfe, and J. E. McGuigan. 1984. "Pentagastrin-stimulated gastric acid secretion by the isolated perfused rat stomach." *Life Sci* 34 (25): 2515-23. https://doi.org/10.1016/0024-3205(84)90289-3.

Soga, J., M. D. Tazawa, and H. Ito. 1969. "Ultrastructural demonstration of specific secretory granules of Mastomys gastric carcinoids." *Acta Med Biol (Niigata)* 17 (2): 119-24.

Solcia, E., C. Capella, R. Fiocca, G. Rindi, and J. Rosai. 1990. "Gastric argyrophil carcinoidosis in patients with Zollinger-Ellison syndrome due to type 1 multiple endocrine neoplasia. A newly recognized association." *Am J Surg Pathol* 14 (6): 503-13.

Soll, A. H. 1982. "Potentiating interactions of gastric stimulants on [14 C] aminopyrine accumulation by isolated canine parietal cells." *Gastroenterology* 83 (1 Pt 2): 216-23.

Sordal, O., G. Qvigstad, I. S. Nordrum, A. K. Sandvik, B. I. Gustafsson, and H. Waldum. 2014. "The PAS positive material in gastric cancer cells of signet ring type is not mucin." *Exp Mol Pathol* 96 (3): 274-8. https://doi.org/10.1016/j.yexmp.2014.02.008.

Tielemans, Y., G. Willems, F. Sundler, and R. Hakanson. 1990. "Self-replication of enterochromaffin-like cells in the mouse stomach." *Digestion* 45 (3): 138-46. https://doi.org/10.1159/000200235.

Uemura, N., S. Okamoto, S. Yamamoto, N. Matsumura, S. Yamaguchi, M. Yamakido, K. Taniyama, N. Sasaki, and R. J. Schlemper. 2001. "Helicobacter pylori infection and the development of gastric cancer." *N Engl J Med* 345 (11): 784-9. https://doi.org/10.1056/NEJMoa001999.

Waldum, H. L., S. Aase, I. Kvetnoi, E. Brenna, A. K. Sandvik, U. Syversen, G. Johnsen, L. Vatten, and J. M. Polak. 1998. "Neuroendocrine differentiation in human gastric carcinoma." *Cancer* 83 (3): 435-44.

Waldum, H. L., J. S. Arnestad, E. Brenna, I. Eide, U. Syversen, and A. K. Sandvik. 1996. "Marked increase in gastric acid secretory capacity after omeprazole treatment." *Gut* 39 (5): 649-53.

Waldum, H. L., B. Bjorvatn, and P. G. Burhol. 1981. "Gastritis, peptic ulcer disease, inflammatory bowel disease, and stomach and colon cancers-are they all caused by viral infections?" *Med Hypotheses* 7 (11): 1329-38. https://doi.org/10.1016/0306-9877(81)90123-7.

Waldum, H. L., and E. Brenna. 1996. "Non-proliferative capacity of endocrine cells of the human gastro-intestinal tract." *Histochem J* 28 (5): 397-8. https://doi.org/10.1007/bf02331403.

Waldum, H. L., E. Brenna, and A. K. Sandvik. 1998. "Maximal gastric acid secretion in man: a concept that needs precision." *Scand J Gastroenterol* 33 (10): 1009-15. https://doi.org/10.1080/003655298750026679.

Waldum, H. L., O. A. Haugen, C. Isaksen, R. Mecsei, and A. K. Sandvik. 1991. "Enterochromaffin-like tumour cells in the diffuse but not the intestinal type of gastric carcinomas." *Eur J Gastroenterol Hepatol* 3: 245-249.

Waldum, H. L., O. Hauso, O. F. Sordal, and R. Fossmark. 2015. "Gastrin May Mediate the Carcinogenic Effect of Helicobacter pylori Infection of the Stomach." *Dig Dis Sci* 60 (6): 1522-7. https://doi.org/10.1007/s10620-014-3468-9.

Waldum, H. L., T. Lehy, E. Brenna, A. K. Sandvik, H. Petersen, B. S. Sognen, S. Bonfils, and M. J. Lewin. 1991. "Effect of the histamine-1 antagonist astemizole alone or with omeprazole on rat gastric mucosa." *Scand J Gastroenterol* 26 (1): 23-35.

Waldum, H. L., K. Oberg, O. F. Sordal, A. K. Sandvik, B. I. Gustafsson, P. Mjones, and R. Fossmark. 2018. "Not only stem cells, but also mature cells, particularly neuroendocrine cells, may develop into tumours: time for a paradigm shift." *Therap Adv Gastroenterol* 11: 1756284818775054. https://doi.org/10.1177/1756284818775054.

Waldum, H. L., A. Sandvik, and E. Brenna. 1993. "Gastrin, the enterochromaffinlike cell, and gastric tumors." *Gastroenterology* 105 (4): 1264-6. https://doi.org/10.1016/0016-5085(93)90990-t.

Waldum, H. L., A. K. Sandvik, E. Brenna, and P. M. Kleveland. 1996. "The gastrin-histamine sequence." *Gastroenterology* 111 (3): 838-9. https://doi.org/10.1053/gast.1996.v111.agast961110838.

Waldum, H. L., A. K. Sandvik, E. Brenna, and B. Schulze Sognen. 1991. "Radioimmunoassay of histamine." *Scand J Gastroenterol Suppl* 180: 32-9.

Wang, T., S. Shigdar, M. P. Gantier, Y. Hou, L. Wang, Y. Li, H. A. Shamaileh, W. Yin, S. F. Zhou, X. Zhao, and W. Duan. 2015. "Cancer stem cell targeted therapy: progress amid controversies." *Oncotarget* 6 (42): 44191-206. https://doi.org/10.18632/oncotarget.6176.

Wilander, E. 1980. "Achylia, pernicious anaemia, ECL cells and gastric carcinoids." *Virchows Arch A Pathol Anat Histol* 387 (3): 371-3.

Will, R. G., J. W. Ironside, M. Zeidler, S. N. Cousens, K. Estibeiro, A. Alperovitch, S. Poser, M. Pocchiari, A. Hofman, and P. G. Smith. 1996.

"A new variant of Creutzfeldt-Jakob disease in the UK." *Lancet* 347 (9006): 921-5. https://doi.org/10.1016/s0140-6736(96)91412-9.
Wormsley, K. G., and M. I. Grossman. 1965. "Maximal histalog test in control subjects and patients with peptic ulcer." *Gut* 6 (5): 427-35. https://doi.org/10.1136/gut.6.5.427.
Zamcheck, N., E. Grable, A. Ley, and L. Norman. 1955. "Occurrence of gastric cancer among patients with pernicious anemia at the Boston City Hospital." *N Engl J Med* 252 (26): 1103-10. https://doi.org/10.1056/nejm195506302522601.
Zollinger, R. M., and E. H. Ellison. 1955. "Primary peptic ulcerations of the jejunum associated with islet cell tumors of the pancreas." *Ann Surg* 142 (4): 709-23; discussion, 724-8.

CHAPTER 4

SPECIAL OBSERVATIONS

Abstract

This chapter describes my experiences with the pharmaceutical industry.

1. In the late eighties, the best scientist in gastric physiology at Astra, Håkan Larsson, was given an administrative position. Considering the many important questions related to PPI treatment, I found this peculiar.
2. We wrote an overview called "Histamine and the Stomach" based on our results on the isolated rat stomach. As I see it, this review is still up to date. Obviously, pharmaceutical companies also found it to be of interest since an English-speaking lawyer came to my office to discuss my point of view and my relationship to pharmaceutical industry. I was only contacted once.
3. In Norway we were encouraged to apply for grants from the European Union (EU). I applied for grants to research gastric cancer and the role of gastric juice in the defense against prion diseases. After the third rejection, which came with particularly humiliating remarks, I concluded that I would not receive EU funding if my work would potentially have negative consequences for European industry.
4. Based upon our studies showing that maximal histamine stimulation exceeded maximal gastrin stimulated acid secretion and that histamine release is dependent upon ECL cell mass, which is regulated by gastrin, it was obvious that PPI treatment had to induce rebound acid secretion, which had been denied until our study. Curiously, our study was met negatively despite PPIs being the most used group of drugs. However, when this point was repeated by one of the initial reviewers, it was mentioned on the front page of *Gastroenterology*.
5. Guidelines are important, particularly for pharmaceutical companies. Astra invited a selected group of gastroenterologists to a meeting on the treatment of gastro-esophageal reflux disease (GERD) where they had prepared questions and answers. The answers were handled

by doctors who had very close connections to Astra, which also helped them when writing the manuscript. It was accepted for publication in the *BMJ*, and I spent a year getting a letter that described how this guideline was biased, published.

6. I was contacted by a representative from FDA at an AGA meeting due to my publication on rebound acid secretion. Some years later, I was invited to participate at a hearing in Washington on over-the-counter PPIs. I was the only expert from Europe, and there were four from North America. I was surprised that one of them was accepted as independent. Nevertheless, over-the-counter PPIs were delayed, but only for a year. Several years later, they were also accepted to be sold over-the-counter in Norway despite my opposition. I believe this to be one of the worst examples of the lack of biological knowledge and respect in clinical medicine.
7. Around 2000, the "Norwegian Research Council" decided to have different research groups evaluated by external committees. I felt that this was positive and thought that our many publications and PhD candidates would give us a high ranking. However, during the oral presentation, I immediately felt a negative atmosphere in the committee, which was dominated by Swedes. We received such a bad rating that it was not worthwhile applying for national grants anymore.
8. About ten years ago I applied for a professorship in Stockholm. The evaluation committee was not able to come to a united conclusion. However, I was given the lowest score in every aspect by two of the members. A new committee was established, and I was awarded second position which was fair.
9. Around 2000, I was invited to participate in a meeting, which considered the predictive value for humans of rodent studies with respect to stomach neuroendocrine tumors. This was organized by the "International Agency for Research on Cancer". The meeting was good, and we were asked to deliver our manuscript for the book within a short time. However, the book did not appear until I contacted the head of WHO more than two years later.
10. The crucial question related to PPI and cancer is the role of hypergastrinemia. Hypergastrinemia was known to induce gastric neuroendocrine tumors in humans before the introduction of PPIs. In addition, PPIs were early recognized to cause tumors in rodents. Nevertheless, the producer was able to convince the scientific community that rodents studies had no relevance for man. Early on,

Astra claimed that there were no more side effects with omeprazole than histamine-2 blockers.

11. My experience with journals has mostly been based on their reluctance to accept papers that have negative consequences for the pharmaceutical industry. However, my letters related to published papers were accepted until fairly recently.
12. In 2011, I wrote a letter together with Public Citizen, Washington, to the FDA about the safety of PPIs. However, a group of American experts denied that there were any problems and nothing more happened.
13. Recently a very large study on the side effects of PPIs was published in *Gastroenterology*, which accompanied by an editorial claiming that the truth had finally been found. The editorial only concentrated on some human studies and did not take animal studies or those on the role of gastrin's target cell (the ECL cell) in human carcinogenesis into consideration. I felt that the editorial was misleading and wrote a letter that was rejected. It is clearly impossible to be open about the side effects of PPIs.

Keywords: acid, animal studies; classification of gastric cancer; ECL cell; evaluations; European Union; FDA; gastric cancer; gastrin; gastro-esophageal reflux disease; histamine 2 blocker; latency; neuroendocrine tumors; pharmaceutical companies; proton pump inhibitors; physiology; scientific journals; side effects.

The move from basic science to administration by Håkan Larsson

During my long clinical and scientific career, I have met scientists from the pharmaceutical industry and universities, including those switching from university to company positions. My impression has been that people go from universities into industry because of the higher wages, but that they also end up disappointed because they lose their scientific freedom.

At the beginning of my career, I was naïve and thought that the pharmaceutical industry and independent scientists had the same final interest: to disclose the truth. Over time, I have realized that the pharmaceutical industry suppresses data that indicates long-term side effects. In the late eighties, Håkan Larsson was the leading experimental scientist in Astra (Larsson et al. 1988), and we cooperated with him (Kleveland, Waldum, and Larsson 1987). He was also one of the opponents to my second PhD candidate, Arne Sandvik. Håkan Larsson was, however, abruptly moved from gastric physiology to Helicobacter pylori and then later to administration. He is to me, an example of a brilliant scientist who was no longer allowed to work on a subject where he could have made a large contribution.

This also exemplifies the fact that that pharmaceutical companies do not want to complete research that can be seen negatively due to its components, even though it is important to human health.

Visit from a lawyer from the US/England

In 1989, I wrote a review for the *Scandinavian Journal of Gastroenterology*, called "Histamine and the stomach" (H. L. Waldum and Sandvik 1989). This was many years ahead of other papers in the field, and this fact has been confirmed in virtually every aspect. Apparently, others also realized the importance of this paper, as I was contacted by a lawyer who wanted to visit me. I was flattered and thought that I might become rich. He appeared at my small office one day. The office was stuffed with papers, and I was not especially elegantly dressed.

As I understood it, he came from abroad just to meet me. During a 30-minute stay, we talked about research and the possibility of working for the pharmaceutical industry. I was not enthusiastic, but nevertheless expressed some interest. When he left, he said that I would be contacted again. However, that never happened. I suspect that he felt that I, and the conditions in which I worked, did not represent any real threat to his company. Therefore, it was not worthwhile trying to buy me out from my position. An alternative explanation is, of course, that he felt that I was not for sale, and therefore it would be dangerous to present me with an offer.

Experience with European Union (EU) applications

In the early nineties, I participated in committees for the Norwegian Research Council, and it became clear to me that Norway spent a lot of money in the EU research system, and that it was important for us to get some of this money back for Norwegian research. During these years, I spent a lot of time preparing applications, albeit with a rather bad rating.

I stopped sending new applications when I not only received a refusal for the third time, but also offensive comments. My applications were related to the role of gastric acid in biology and the possible danger of drug induced hypoacidity with secondary hypergastrinemia. Moreover, my last EU application was on the role of gastric juice in the defense against prion diseases, which was not considered to be of importance. However, recent findings suggest that gut infection is the cause of neurodegenerative diseases (Prusiner 2012), particularly Parkinson′s disease (Liddle 2018), and so perhaps our application was not so bad?

Considering the increasingly high use of PPIs, I felt that that these issues should be of interest. However, I realized that the EU would not support work that was potentially harmful to its own pharmaceutical industry, and that the system was heavily influenced by economic interests. From that point, I have been happy that Norway is not a full member of the EU, which has a bad reputation with corruption in general.

Rebound acid hypersecretion and my experiences with *The Lancet*, *Nature Medicine*, and the Digestive Disease Week (DDW) congress

When we demonstrated that omeprazole induced a marked hypersecretion of gastric acid when it was given in ordinary clinical doses for three months (H. L. Waldum et al. 1996), I immediately felt that this was why problems occurred when stopping treatment (Bjornsson 2011).

Taking into consideration that PPIs are among the most widely used drugs and have now started to be given to patients with dyspepsia (Talley et al. 1998), we realized the potential clinical importance of our findings. We therefore sent the manuscript to *The Lancet*. After a few months, we received a refusal based upon four referee reports: two were very positive but the others did not find anything of interest in it. The two negative reports came up with irrelevant arguments and, in addition, they claimed that we had not studied enough patients. However, we had studied ten patients with an acid secretion test, prior to starting and two weeks after a 3-months treatment period, and the hypersecretion was highly significant. I sent a letter to the editor, arguing that there was no basis for the negative reports, and that the p-value showed that we had examined enough patients. However, the editor stuck to his decision, and three years later one of the positive reviewers copied our study and published it in *Gastroenterology* (Gillen et al. 1999).

We then sent our manuscript to *GUT* but even this journal hesitated. Why should scientific journals be afraid of publishing manuscripts with negative consequences to pharmaceutical companies? Manuscripts should be only judged by their scientific and clinical importance. During my career, I have often heard that this is controversial. I have always believed that "controversial" is a word that has nothing to do with science.

Digestive Disease Week (DDW) is held during the spring. In 1996, I submitted an abstract on rebound acid hypersecretion after the use of PPIs to them. The pharmaceutical industry makes a significant financial contribution to this meeting and, at that time, Astra was the largest sponsor. I suppose that this is the reason why I have never been allowed to orally

present my work there. I have attended 35 meetings and often sent abstracts, but this has become less frequent in recent years. Nevertheless, my abstract was accepted for a poster presentation, but given a late slot on the last day of the meeting with no time to discuss the results and, in addition, many people had already left at this point.

However, just before taking down my poster, I was contacted by a person from the Food and Drug Administration (FDA). He was very interested in our work, and he later invited me to the FDA meeting on over-the-counter PPI in Washington in 2000, which I will discuss in more detail shortly. On one of the first days of the DDW meeting, there was an oral presentation with some relevance to rebound acid secretion. I participated heavily in the debate, and the editor of *GUT* decided to accept our manuscript on rebound acid hypersecretion after hearing me speak. My experience from the handling of that manuscript, supported and strengthened my conviction regarding the difficulties in publishing studies with negative consequences for industrial companies.

The importance of rebound acid hypersecretion after using PPIs was doubted by the scientific community. We did another study showing that PPI treatment increased tolerance to histamine-2 blockers (Qvigstad et al. 1998), which should have influenced clinical practice so that patients with milder forms of reflux esophagitis, and particularly those with reflux symptoms without esophagitis, were given histamine-2 blockers as an initial treatment.

Based upon our belief that PPI treatment could be harmful, we hesitated to start a study to find out whether giving PPIs to healthy volunteers for a period of time could induce dyspeptic symptoms. Fortunately, a Danish group (Reimer et al. 2009) studied healthy medical students, which showed that they had developed dyspepsia the week after stopping the PPI treatment. This renewed the interest in gastric acid hypersecretion. Even *Nature* found the subject of interest, and I was contacted by telephone and interviewed.

I was greatly surprised when I read the resulting article in the journal, as only McColl (the man who copied my study) was cited. I also need to mention that I was then contacted by *Nature* some years later and interviewed by one of their journalists. The interview was mailed to me, and I corrected it but I did not hear anything afterwards, and it was not published.

It is understandable that not everything a journalist comes up with gets published, but I would expect a note to be sent to those who have spent time working on an article.

It is also peculiar that there have been meta-analyses of published studies, which have been performed in such a way that rebound acid hypersecretion would not be expected to occur (Hunfeld, Geus, and Kuipers 2007). Therefore, the conclusion was that rebound acid hypersecretion after the use of PPIs was not important. In general, this meta-analysis demonstrates the weakness in this evaluation form.

UNIVERSITETET I TRONDHEIM
DET MEDISINSKE FAKULTET
Medisinsk avdeling
Gastroenterologisk seksjon

Vår saksbehandler, tlf.

27.11.95

Vår dato - referanse
19.03.99 HLW/bm
Deres dato - referanse

Editor Richard Horton
The Lancet
42 Bedford Square
LONDON WC1B 3SL
UK

Dear Sir,

Re. Manuscript 95/9405

Thank you for the evaluation of the manuscript *Marked increase in gastric acid secretory capacity in patients with reflux oesophagitis after a tree months period with a proton pump inhibitor in a conventional dose.*

In my accompanying letter I asked you not to send the manuscript for evaluation to any researcher with connection to any pharmaceutical company producing proton pump inhibitor. The reason for writing that was that I have experienced during the last five to ten years that the influence of pharmaceutical companies on medical science has increased in a way making it difficult to publish manuscripts with negative consequences for pharmaceutical companies.

Of course I am confident that the Editorial Board of The Lancet is independent. However, the affiliation between researchers and pharmaceutical companies is naturally not obvious for editors. Among the four reviewers that evaluated our manuscript, I feel that two of them, whom I call reviewer B and C, have made comments that make me sceptical concerning their scientific independence. I therefore will make comments on all the suggestions and remarks of the reviewers in the hope that the Editorial Board will evaluate the manuscript together with the enclosed letter and reconsider the decision not to publish it.

Reviewer A

This reviewer was generally positive to our work. He states that the design of the study was appropriate. However, he makes a negative remark concerning the number of patients included, and that it was made as an open study.

Our study did not include any subjective data, so it should obviously not be necessary to do it as a blinded study. The number of patients included was quite sufficient as shown by the highly significant results obtained. It should be realized that it is not necessary to include a huge number of patients to disclose marked differences. The reviewer refers to a previous study showing no rebound acid hypersecretion in healthy volunteers after a three weeks treatment period with omeprazole 40 mg daily. As quoted by the reviewer the treatment period was probably too short to disclose acid hypersecretion. It should be realized that the acid hypersecretion after treatment with proton pump inhibitors is not due to any up or down regulation of receptors, but just due to the trophic effect of hypergastrinemia on the ECL cell. Since it takes time to develop a significant ECL cell hyperplasia a longer treatment period is needed.

Concerning Helicobacter pylori and our results, the manuscript has been changed according to the suggestions made by the reviewer. With regard to the detailed comments by the reviewer A we think that figure 1 clarifies the design of the study, but of course it could be deleted.

Besøksadresse/Location:
Olav Kyrresgt. 17

Postadresse/Address:
Regionsykehuset i Trondheim
N-7006 Trondheim

University of Trondheim
Faculty of Medicine
Department of Medicine
Section of Gastroenterology
Int. phone : +47 73 59 74 63
Int. fax : +47 73 59 75 46

DET MEDISINSKE FAKULTET 19-03-99

We feel, however, that omitting figure 2 will make the interpretation for the reader more difficult. After all, most clinicians do know something about the normal gastrin values whereas an integrated two-hour response is not so easily interpreted.

We do, however, agree that the patients positive for Helicobacter pylori should be identified on the figures, which has been done.

Point 4. Basal gastric acid secretion has been determined for decades and it does not seem appropriate to me to delete it. After all, the ratio between basal and maximal acid secretion is an important parameter in for example the diagnosis of Zollinger Ellison syndrome.

Conclusion
This referee was generally positive to our manuscript, and has made some suggestions which we have followed and which have improved the manuscript.

Reviewer B
The comments made by this reviewer made me doubt this reviewers scientific standard or independence. This reviewer claims that an increase in pentagastrin stimulated acid secretion from a mean of 29.7 to 44.8 mmol/h is not great. This is a 50 % increase and is at least as much as the increase in gastric acid secretory capacity in patients with duodenal ulcer compared with normal subjects. This reviewer seems to be unaware of the large amount of literature and work done during many decades. He also seems to be unaware of older studies showing that maximal acid secretion is rather constant in the individual patient (White & Juniper, Dig Dis 1973,18,7-13). He also asks for data on H_2-blockers. This is to me a typical example of how to try to stop a manuscript by asking for other data which at the first glance seems appropriate. Studies on acid rebound after H_2-blockers were done as early as in the late seventies. Thus, a six week course of oral cimetidine did not affect pentagastrin stimulated acid secretion (Aadland et al., Scand J Gastroenterol 1978,13,193-197). The new important finding of the present study is that protonpump inhibitors do induce gastric acid hypersecretion, and it seems quite unnecessary to demand a comparison with H_2- blockers which have been thoroughly examined for rebound acid hypersecretion previously.

The next phrase in the comments from this reviewer is quite remarkable: *«If it is assumed that treatment for oesophagitis is required and that acid suppression is necessary for adequate treatment, the findings of this study may just reflect a necessary consequence of successful treatment of reflux oesophagitis».* What does this mean? I do feel that this sentence clearly shows the scientific attitude of this reviewer. Again, the reviewer ask for comparative data with H_2- receptor antagonists which I have referred to above.

It is also typically asked for the clinical consequences. Actually our manuscript open up for new studies to determine the clinical consequences of our findings. Our study gives the argument for doing new studies on the clinical consequences of post-treatment acid hypersecretion.

Concerning the minor comments, we will change the manuscript according to suggestions 1 and 2. The biopsies were assessed blindly. Serology was used for Helicobacter pylori diagnosis since we did not take any biopsy from the antrum for Helicobacter pylori diagnosis.

Point 5. The correct is mmol.
Point 6. The figure will be changed as suggested
Point 7. It is better to give the data for the individual patients and thus allow the reader direct access to the original data, than using mean values

Side 2

Reviewer C
This reviewer suggests that we did a lot of comparisons for many parameters and included the parameters that we found to be significantly different. Therefore, he asks for Bonferroni correction.

I do hope that the Editorial Board does not pay too much consideration on this reviewers statement since he actually criticizes the manuscript on the basis of a false presumption. Of course the parameters studied were based upon our knowledge of the regulation of gastric acid secretion and we have not examined any other parameters than those reported in the manuscript. The data for the individual patient are given in the figures 2 and 3 and table 2. These clearly shows that the results are clear-cut with or without statistical evaluation.

We feel that this reviewer has not been able to give any argument of importance against the manuscript or the results presented.

Reviewer D
Reviewer D is generally positive towards the manuscript. Among the major comments this reviewer has given, the argument concerning basal and food-stimulated acid output may be easily answered. Actually, we showed in the present study that basal acid secretion was increased. Moreover, it is well known that gastrin is the dominant secretagogue (actually 90 %) of meal-stimulated acid secretion (Blair et al., Gastroenterology 1987,92,944-949). Therefore, it is no doubt that the recorded findings have implications for gastric acidity in vivo. This reviewer also asks for studies on gastric acid secretion following gastrin releasing peptide (GRP). This comment has some relevance. However, GRP is not available for patient treatment, only as a chemical substance. Moreover, GRP-stimulated acid secretion depends on the G-cell mass, the ECL cell mass and the parietal cell mass whereas pentagastrin-stimulated acid secretion only depends on the ECL cell and the parietal cell masses. Since drug induced hypo-/anacidity also increases the G-cell mass (Creutzfeldt et al., Digestion 1986,35(suppl 1),84-97), it would be expected that GRP and meal-stimulated acid secretion would be even more enhanced than pentagastrin-stimulated acid secretion.

I do not, however, think that it is fair to use those arguments against our manuscript. After all we have shown without doubt that omeprazole treatment induces rebound gastric acid hypersecretion. In further studies I do agree that GRP-stimulated acid secretion could be examined as well as pentagastrin-stimulated acid secretion. To me this is hardly an argument against, but more in favour of our manuscript.

Conclusion
We have for the first time, demonstrated gastric acid rebound hypersecretion after a treatment period with a protonpump inhibitor. The reason why this has not been demonstrated before is that most researchers have not understood that the ECL cell plays a central role in the regulation of gastric acid secretion (Waldum et al., Gut 1991,32,698-701), and that the ECL cell mass is a limiting factor in gastric acid secretion (Waldum & Sandvik, Scand J Gastroenterol 1989,24,330-339). Moreover, this increase in gastric acid secretory capacity is based on the trophic effect on the ECL cell and not on upregulation of receptors. Therefore, the treatment period needs to be of sufficient length to induce a detectable increase in acid secretory capacity. It is probable that the demonstrated increase in gastric acid secretory capacity has important clinical consequences, which after our study obviously need to be studied. The pharmaceutical industry is now trying to induce treatment with protonpump inhibitors not only on patients with reflux oesophagitis, but also in «patients» with heartburn , a symptom which affects 10 - 30 % of the population (see enclosed program from a recent meeting).

I am firmly of the opinion that the reviewers have not given any important comments against our study. We have disclosed an important side effect of drugs that are commonly used. Furthermore, I will question the scientific independence of two of the reviewers. I therefore hope that the Editorial Board after having seen my comments, will re-evaluate the paper and hopefully change the decision not to publish it. I am sure that the results of our study are of

DET MEDISINSKE FAKULTET 19-03-99

general importance justifying it to be published in The Lancet. Moreover, I have confidence in the Editorial Board in The Lancet (there are, however, many journals that I would not even think of sending this paper to), which have dealt with the problem of corruption in academic institutions quite recently (Lancet 1993,342,315-316).

I do hope that you can make a decision within two weeks.

Sincerely yours

Helge L. Waldum
Professor of Medicine

Enclosure:
- Program from a recent meeting on heart-burn
- Editorial. The Lancet 1993,342,315-316: Are academic institutions corrupt?
- Comments from the reviewers
- Modified manuscript (the manuscript is changed according to some of the suggestions of the reviewers (marked *))

Side 4

NTNU
Norwegian University of
Science and Technology

Faculty of Medicine
Department of Intra-Abdominal Diseases

KOPI

Editor Richard Horton
The Lancet
42 Bedford Square
LONDON WC1B 3SL
UK

Our consultant:
Telephone no.:

Dated:	Our ref.:	Your letter dated:	Your ref.:
1999-04-13	HLW/bm		

Dear Sir,

Re. Manuscript 95/9405

In 1995 I sent you a manuscript showing a marked rebound acid hypersecretion after omeprazole treatment. I was very astonished by your reviewers of whom two were very positive whereas the other two could not find anything positive at all. It was very difficult to understand why the views of the reviewers could be so different. In a letter afterwards I could show that the arguments of the two negative reviewers were not relevant at all. Nevertheless, you did not accept the manuscript. It was, however, accepted in Gut and now similar findings have been reported in Gastroenterology and quoted on the front page of Gastroenterology.

I felt, and still feel, that it was difficult to understand how the two negative reviewers had "fabricated" negative aspects with our study. It is reason to believe that links to pharmaceutical industry can influence medical scientists. This is indeed an important question, and with the appearance of an article in Gastroenterology completely confirming our results, I find reason to write to you again and I hope that you will publish and make a comment to our letter in The Lancet. I enclose the front page and the article published in Gastroenterology. Furthermore, I enclose our publication in Gut.

Sincerely yours,

Helge L. Waldum
Professor of Medicine

Enclosure.

Address
Regionsykehuset i Trondheim
N-7006 Trondheim
Norway

Location
Olav Kyrres g. 17
Regionsykehuset i Trondheim

Tel. +47 73 86 85 60
Fax +47 73 86 75 46
Org. no. NO 974 767 880

NTNU
Norwegian University of Science and Technology

Faculty of Medicine
Department of Intra-Abdominal Diseases

Senior Editor Stephanie Clark, Ph.D.
The Lancet
42 Bedford Square
LONDON WC1B 3SL
UK

Telephone no.:

Dated:	Our ref.:	Your letter dated:	Your ref.:
1999-12-20	HLW/bm	1999-06-18	SC/DCB-L9/2455

Dear Stephanie Clark,

In April 1999 I sent you a letter concerning a manuscript that I had submitted to The Lancet in 1995. The manuscript no. 95/9405 was evaluated by four reviewers, and two of them gave comments that either demonstrated lack of knowledge of the area or non-scientific reasons for finding arguments against the manuscript. Our manuscript was later published in Gut, and in 1999 our study was reproduced and published in Gastroenterology. Since I had a correspondence with the Editor of The Lancet in 1995 about the rejection of our manuscript, I found it natural to send a letter for publication in The Lancet regarding the handling of this manuscript. The reason was of course to focus on the peer-review system. In your answer of 18 June 1999, you did to my surprise not deal with this issue at all, but in stead refused my letter claiming that it was not related to The Lancet at all.

When reading the enclosed letter in Science about *Peer Review under Review*, I again thought about the way my manuscript was handled in The Lancet in 1995, and about the formal and arrogant way by which my letter in 1999 was refused. It made me think that there is no will in The Lancet to take a discussion on this issue. I therefore write to you again, hoping that you at least will give an answer with appropriate comments on the issue that I have raised.

Sincerely yours

Helge L. Waldum
Professor of Medicine

Enclosure.

Address	Location	Tel. +47 73 86 85 60	Page 1 of 1
Regionsykehuset i Trondheim	Olav Kyrres g. 17	Fax +47 73 86 75 46	clark, s. lancet, 15.12.
N-7006 Trondheim	Regionsykehuset i Trondheim	Org. no. NO 974 767 880	
Norway			

Letter to the Editor in *Aliment Pharmacol Ther* (rejected)

Dear Sir.

Rebound acid hypersecretion

We red the paper" Systematic review: rebound acid hypersecretion after therapy with proton pump inhibitors "by Hunfeld et al [1] with great interest. The authors based their review on eight studies where proton pump inhibitors (PPIs) were given at accepted clinical doses from 1 to 90 days and described no rebound acid hypersecretion (RAHS) in 5 studies where the patients/subjects were treated from 1 to 25 days and RAHS in 3 studies where the treatment duration was from 56 to 90 days. From these data they concluded that there is no strong evidence for a clinically relevant increased acid production after withdrawal of PPI therapy.[1]

The occurance of RAHS after administration of PPI was first demonstrated in the rat after 3 months of omeprazole administration[2]. Later, the same phenomenon was found in humans having used PPI for 90 days [3] and after 56 days[4, 5].
As regards possible mechanisms that could explain RAHS after cessation of proton pump inhibition, there is evidence that an increase in the enterochromaffin-like (ECL) cell population caused by long term hypergastrinemia is of importance[3, 6]. In the rat we have shown that the gastrin-stimulated histamine release is dependent of the ECL cell mass [7], and it is well-known that hypergastrinemia secondary to gastric hypoacidity is a natural consequence of PPI treatment, resulting in ECL cell hyperplasia[8]. Two years ago we published in "Alimentary Pharmacolocy and Therapeutics" a study that showed an increase in pentagastrin stimulatied acid secretion 4 and 8 weeks after cessation of long-term PPI-use compared with 16 and 26 weeks [6]. There was a reduction in histidine decarboxylase positive cells (ECL cells) in biopsies from the oxyntic mucosa 26 weeks after cessation compared with during PPI treatment [6].
As it takes time to develop significant ECL cell hyperplasia , it is not possible to evaluate PPI-induced RAHS after one single dose, nor after 25 days use, although the studies had a randomized design.
According to Hunfeld et al the studies where PPI was administered for 1-25 days provide evidence grade A2 or B that RAHS does not occur after PPI use, whereas we would claim that these five studies merely show that PPI must be used more than 1-25 days to induce RAHS. This issue is mentioned in the discussion part of the review but it does not influence the authours conclusions. Moreover, we think conclusions about the existance of RAHS should not be based on studies that due to the study design could not possibly demonstrate RAHS.

In conclusion, both physiological and statistical knowledge is needed when reviewing RASH and at present it is meaningless to apply a meta-analysis on this biological phenomenon.

References:

1 Hunfeld N, Geus W, Kuipers EJ. Systematic review: rebound acid hypersecretion after therapy with proton pump inhibitors. *Aliment Pharmacol Ther* 2007; **25**: 39-46.

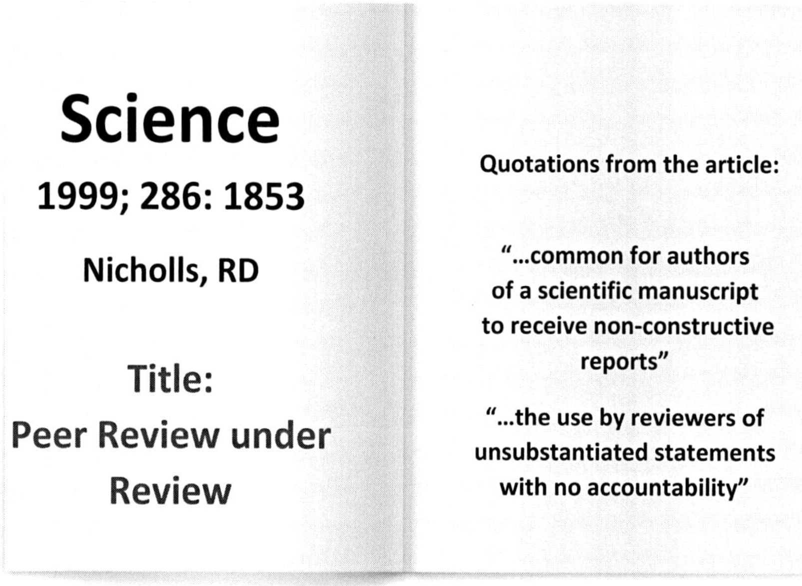
Science
1999; 286: 1853
Nicholls, RD
Title:
Peer Review under Review
Quotations from the article:
"...common for authors of a scientific manuscript to receive non-constructive reports"
"...the use by reviewers of unsubstantiated statements with no accountability"

NTNU
Norwegian University of Science and Technology

Faculty of Medicine
Department of Intra-Abdominal Diseases

KOPI

Editor Daniel K. Podolsky, M.D.
Gastroenterology
AGA National Office
7910 Woodmont Avenue, 7th Floor
Bethesda, Maryland 20814

Our consultant:

Telephone no.:

Dated:	Our ref.:	Your letter dated:	Your ref.:
1999-04-08	HLW/bm		

Dear Sir,

Re: Manuscript No. 99-3411-00

Thank you for your letter of March 31, 1999, concerning our manuscript entitled "The safety of profound acid inhibition".

Of course, I do not agree with you that the clinical impact of the role of the ECL cell in human gastric carcinogenesis has received sufficient attention. *Gastroenterology* has always published papers concluding that profound acid inhibition is safe, and is obviously not yet ready to publish papers with a different view. From a strictly scientific point of view it would have been appropriate to publish the manuscript that you referred to in the letter, claiming that profound acid inhibition was without risk together with ours, and so let the clinicians make the decision how to treat the patients. Of course, with time we will know what view is correct.

In any way, thank you for accepting my letter no. 99-3387-00.

Sincerely yours,

Helge L. Waldum
Professor of Medicine

Address
N-7006 Trondheim
Norway

Location
Olav Kyrres g. 17
Regionsykehuset i Trondheim

Tel. +47 73 86 85 60
Fax +47 73 86 75 46
Org. no. NO 974 767 880

Gastroenterology February 1999, volume 116; Number 2. Front page title: **«Rebound hypersecretion after omeprazole»**	***Gastroenterology*** 1999; 116:239–247 Derek Gillen, Angela A. Wirz, Joy E. Erdill and Kenneth E.L. McCall Title of article: **"Rebound hypersecretion after omeprazole and its relation to on-treatment acid suppression and Helicobacter pylori status."**

The authors followed our research (*Gut* 1996; 39:649-653) and studied gastric acid secretion before and 2 weeks after an 8-week treatment period with omeprazole and confirmed our finding that it induced a substantial increase in acid secretion in Helicobacter negative subjects.

THE LANCET

42 Bedford Square
London WC1B 3SL
United Kingdom

Editor: Richard Horton
Deputy Editor: David Sharp

TEL +44 (0)171 436 4981
FAX +44 (0)171 323 6441

www.thelancet.com

Please quote ref : SC/DCB - L9/2455

18 June 1999

Dr Helge L Waldum
Department of Intra-Abdominal Disease
Faculty of Medicine NTNU
Norwegian University of Science and Technology
Regionsykehuset i Trondheim
N-7006 Trondheim
NORWAY

FAX: 00 47 7 997546

Dear Dr Waldum

Thank you for your letter which we received here on 5 May 1999. I am afraid that our decision is against publication. We have nearly 3000 letters a year submitted for our correspondence section, most of which comment on work that we have published in this journal. Obviously, we have to award priority to those letters.

I am sorry that I cannot be more helpful.

Yours sincerely

Stephanie Clark PhD
Senior Editor

U.S. Agent for The Lancet, 655 Avenue of the Americas, New York NY 10010
The Lancet Publishing Group, a division of Elsevier Science Ltd.
Registered office: The Boulevard, Langford Lane, Kidlington, OX5 1GB. Registered in England No. [illegible]

From: Alisa Opar
To: helge.waldum@medisin.ntnu.no
Subject: Re: Nature Medicine article on proton pump inhibitor therapy
Date: 15. juni 2009 04:53:03

Dear Dr. Waldum,

It was good to talk to you last week. I am pasting your quotes below. Please take a look, and send me any comments by 7am, New York time on Tuesday, June 16.

Best,
Alisa

"I was very pleased when I saw this paper," says Helge Waldum, a gastrointestinal researcher at the Norwegian University of Science and Technology. "Every clinician knows that the patients we put on PPI become more or less dependent. I always suspected that was do to rebound acid hypersecretion; this paper shows how the patients become dependent on the treatment."

"Traditionally, we've used the histamine-2 blockers," says Waldum. "They weren't as efficient as PPIs, but most people who take the histamine-2 blocker are relieved of their symptoms. But then it became convenient to start with PPIs immediately. I believe you should take away as little as possible from normal physical functions, because I think that there are reasons that we have gastric acid. I think that we should start with H2 blockers, and only the patients with the most problems should be put on PPIs."

> On Tue, Jun 9, 2009 at 8:28 AM, Alisa Opar<alisaopar@gmail.com> wrote:
>> Dear Dr. Waldum,
>>
>> I'm writing a news story for the July issue of Nature Medicine on
>> proton pump inhibitors and concerns about potential side effects, like
>> bone fractures, pneumonia, etc. I'm also looking at a study being
>> published in the July issue of Gastroenterology that found evidence
>> that PPI therapy induces the symptoms it's used to treat (attached;
>> under embargo until July 1).
>>
>> Could you take some time to talk about the importance of the paper and
>> this topic this week? My deadline is Friday, June 12, 6pm EDT. Please
>> suggest a couple of days/times that work for you, and the best phone
>> number to reach you. The interview shouldn't take more than 30
>> minutes. Please let me know if you would prefer to answer a few
>> questions via email.
>>
>> Best regards,
>> Alisa Opar
>> 212-979-3143
>> New York, NY
>>
>

> minutes. Please let me know if you would prefer to answer a few
> questions via email.
>
> Best regards,
> Alisa Opar
> 212-979-3143
> New York, NY

From: Helge Waldum
To: Alisa Opar
Subject: Re: Nature Medicine article on proton pump inhibitor therapy

---

Dear Alisa Opar.
I read the news in Nature Medicine but could not see that I was
mentioned. This is a little sad since I was the first to describe
rebound acid hypersecretion after PPItreatment,
and I have always claimed that the patients become physical dependent of
PPI due to this phenomenon. We detected this rebound hypersecretion
due to our animal studies
where we showed that gastrin stimulated acid secretion (and therefore
also meal stimulated acid secretion) depended on gastrin stimulated
histamine release from the ECL cells.
Since histamine release also depends on the ECL cell mass which in turn
is regulated by 24 h gastrin levels, hypergastrinemia which is the
consequence of reduced gastric acidity, will necessary
lead to rebound acid hypersecretion which we showed in 1996. It was,
however, difficult to get that article accepted. I knew that our
finding was important and sent it to " Lancet" where four reviewers
evaluated the paper- two were very positive whereas the other two did
not find any interest at all in the manuscript. The manuscript was
therefore refused in spite of describing (or perhaps therefore)
an important side effect with the most sold drug at that time. I have
since that time claimed that the patients become more dyspeptic after
PPI use due to rebound acid hypersecretion,and have also
suspected that the reason why reflux oesophagitis and anti antireflux
surgery have increased during the last decades are due to PPI treatment.
Because of ethical considerations, we have not done any
study on healthy individuals as the Danish study, which not surprisingly
confirms that individuals become dyspeptic due to such treatment (we
mean that there is a theoretical risk with a period with anacidity
and hypergastrinemia (cancer and infections))
To conclude, during a twenty-year period I have done studies supporting
my view that there are negative consequences related to PPI treatment. I
have been fought by most experts, many of which having a too close
connection
to pharmaceutical companies. Now, when the truth becomes more difficult
to suppress, they try to keep me out of focus. I am sorry to say that I
feel that your omission of my name in your report
is in line with this.
Finally I will add that McColl was one of the two positive reviewers of
my manuscript in "Lancet" and he followed our study exactly and
confirmed our results in his study which he published three years later.
It seems nevertheless a little odd that the original work should not be
focused on.
I expect you to answer this mail
Sincerely
Helge Waldum

Dear Dr. Waldum,
> I'm writing a news story for the July issue of Nature Medicine on
> proton pump inhibitors and concerns about potential side effects, like
> bone fractures, pneumonia, etc. I'm also looking at a study being
> published in the July issue of Gastroenterology that found evidence
> that PPI therapy induces the symptoms it's used to treat (attached;
> under embargo until July 1).
>
> Could you take some time to talk about the importance of the paper and
> this topic this week? My deadline is Friday, June 12, 6pm EDT. Please
> suggest a couple of days/times that work for you, and the best phone
> number to reach you. The interview shouldn't take more than 30

Pentagastrin removed from the market

It is also provoking that pentagastrin, which has been used to assess stimulated acid secretion since the sixties (Gregory and Tracy 1961), has recently become unavailable. Therefore, it is no longer possible to do studies like ours, which showing rebound hypersecretion after the use of PPIs. The production of pentagastrin was stopped, I suppose, because the demand for it was so low, as gastric acid secretory studies are seldom done any more. Perhaps the reduced possibility of performing these types of studies was an intended side effect when stopping its production?

Guidelines for gastro-esophageal reflux disease

Guidelines have become increasingly popular in medicine, and may be of help, particularly for young doctors. However, guidelines formulated as a rule in so-called consensus meetings among a group of experts, may have such a strong impact that they may not allow any deviation.

It is of great importance for a pharmaceutical company to have its product(s) among the options suggested in these guidelines. Moreover, these studies enable the pharmaceutical industry to set the boundaries for the decisions and the resulting guidelines. By relying on so-called evidence-based medicine, the guidelines are regarded as being scientific. However, few seem to consider the fact that the evidence is at best valid only for the study period, which often only lasts a few months.

Therefore, long-term side effects are not taken into consideration and instead decisions are made based upon short-term human studies. Previously, general biological knowledge and long-term animal studies were required prior to their use in humans. In this respect, there was a change when PPIs were accepted for clinical use despite causing malignant tumors in their target organ in rodents.

Glaxo stopped the development of their long-term inhibitor of acid secretion, loxtidine (Poynter et al. 1986), because it created similar tumors to the first PPI, omeprazole. Since omeprazole has been accepted for clinical use, there seems to have been a change in that toxicity in animals is no longer immediately acknowledged to have consequences for humans.

One often hears expressions like “rats are not men”. Taking into consideration that the rat is more than 90% genetically like man, those claiming important species differences should prove why the findings in animals are not of importance to man, rather than the other way around. Additionally, from a commercial point of view, guidelines are important.

It was, therefore, important for Astra to publish guidelines for the treatment of gastro-esophageal reflux disease that advocated PPI treatment in a prestigious journal (Dent et al. 2001). The four authors had very tight connections to Astra and other producers of PPIs, which evident from the list of competing interests. Moreover, Astra had provided funding for the preparation of the manuscript. Thus, there is no doubt that the authors were too closely connected to the PPI companies. The data upon which the guidelines were based, was even more problematic since Astra had invited a "dedicated" group of doctors to the meeting (Genval, Belgium).

Astra had prepared questions, and the participants were given selected alternatives. The answers were collected and served as a basis for the guidelines. Thus, the company had selected the participants, the questions, the possible answers, and engaged some of their closely connected doctors to develop guidelines with assistance of the company itself. I can understand that the company did this because it would certainly increase their profit margins. What is much more problematic, is that the *BMJ* accepted it for publication. The *BMJ* has been regarded as a “clean” journal, but it is impossible to avoid the impression that non-scientific matters were involved when this manuscript was accepted. So many aspects of the article would have obviously made any editor aware that it was biased.

I immediately wrote a letter where I questioned the connection between the pharmaceutical company and the development of these guidelines, and it was accepted within a week. However, the letter did not appear in the journal. When I contacted the editor, I was told that it would be published soon. After a few more months, the response changed as they stated that my letter had to be evaluated legally before it could be published. In other words, the journal had published guidelines on a prevalent disease where the leading pharmaceutical company within the field had been involved in every phase of the process without finding this problematic, but found it difficult to publish a short letter calling attention to these facts. I responded that I would send my letter to an English newspaper if it was not published immediately. It was published nearly one year after it was first accepted (H. L. Waldum and Brenna 2002). The experience with this case showed that even highly reputable old British journals appear to be affected by corruption (see the below correspondence). Interestingly, and perhaps paradoxically, the *BMJ* published an editorial on the problem in 2011 (Gale 2011) with the heading, “Conflict of interest in guideline panel members. A change in the culture of medicine is needed; legislation is not enough." This problem has also been addressed in *Science* (Nicholls 1999).

BMJ

British Medical Journal
BMA House
Tavistock Square
London
WC1H 9JR

www.bmj.com

Intl: +44 020 7387 4499
Tel: 020 7387 4499
Fax: 020 7383 6418
Direct:

Professor L. Waldum
Faculty of Medicine
Dept of Intra-Abdominal Diseases
NTNU
Regionsykehuset i Trondheim
N-7006 Trondheim
Norway

14 May 2001

Dear Professor Waldum

Re Letter to editor Ref: 11335

I am writing in reply to your letter of 27th April, 2001 concerning your response to the article by Dent et al published in our February 10, 2001 issue.

Your letter has been accepted for publication and should appear in a future edition of the journal.

Please accept our apologies for the length of time this is taking. The reason for the delay is that we receive hundreds of letters each week and as a result, letters have to wait for an available slot in the paper journal. Your letter is with the technical editors at the present time so I anticipate that it will only be a few weeks now before it is published.

Best wishes
Yours sincerely

Janet Cross
Editorial Assistant
jcross@bmj.com

Re: Letter to editor Ref: 11335

Subject: Re: Letter to editor Ref: 11335
Date: Wed, 26 Sep 2001 09:37:54 +0100
From: "Janet Cross" <jcross@bmj.com>
To: Berit Myren <Berit.Myren@medisin.ntnu.no>

Dear Prof Waldum
I have forwarded your email to Sharon Davies, letters editor who decides when letters can be published. I'm sorry for the delay in replying but I have been away and just returned today.
Thank you
Janet Cross

Berit Myren wrote:

> **From, Professor Helge L. Waldum**
>
> **Letter to editor Ref: 11335**
>
> Dear Janet Cross,
>
> My letter related to a published article in February and was accepted on 14 May 2001. In the letter of acceptance it was apologised for the time taking for handling it, and it was stated that the letter was anticipated to appear within a few weeks. Since I have not seen the letter yet in your journal, and I have not received any proof of the letter, I hereby send you this e-mail to have more exact information of the time of appearance. I would also remind you on my later e-mail concerning the heading of the letter.
>
> Sincerely yours
> Helge L. Waldum
> Professor of Medicine

Re: Letter to editor Ref: 11335

Subject: **Re: Letter to editor Ref: 11335**
Date: Mon, 17 Dec 2001 14:49:39 +0000
From: "Janet Cross" <jcross@bmj.com>
To: Berit Myren <Berit.Myren@medisin.ntnu.no>

Dear Professor Waldum
Thank you for your enquiry.
I am very sorry that your letter has still not been published.
Decisions as to when letters are published are made by the letters editor, Sharon Davies.I regret that I have no control or authority in this regard but I will forward your email on to her.
Many thanks
Janet Cross
Letters.

Berit Myren wrote:

> **From Professor Helge L. Waldum:**
>
> Letter to editor Ref: 11335
>
> Dear Janet Cross,
>
> Since I have not heard from you after our two agreeable telephone talks during the last two monts, I am again sending you an e-mail to hear at what time my letter will appear in BMJ. I do understand that you have problems how to handle this task, which I must say is solely due to bad judgement by the journal. If you have problems to give an answer to my letter, why not just publish my letter without comments and let the readers make their own judgement?
>
> Sincerely yours
> Helge L. Waldum
> Professor of Medicine

Sendt 22.01 file:///Untitlec

From Professor Helge L. Waldum

Dear Sharon Davies,

I will not have my letter published in an electronic way because as I answered nearly one year ago, I wanted to reach the same readers that read the original article by Dent and co-workers. I certainly not want to withdraw a letter that has been accepted eight months ago, and in the letter acceptance it was apologised for the length of time in accepting it. It is difficult for me to understand why publishing the letter should be handled in the ethics committee. In my mind I think that what you should discuss in such a meeting is the relationship between BMJ and pharmaceutical companies. It is obvious that you have accepted a publication with direct guidelines for drug treatment for a large proportion of patients based upon biased data and biased treatment of these data.

In conclusion, my letter has been accepted for publication in BMJ. If it had not been accepted for publication in BMJ, I would have gone public with my letter since it obviously discloses a connection between your journal and commercial interests. The editor of the journal must be able himself to decide when to publish an accepted letter. It seems to me that BMJ has tried to avoid the publishing of the letter because it is embarrassing for the journal, hoping that I would forget it and later claim that is was too late to publish it.

Sincerely yours
Helge L. Waldum
Professor of Medicine

Sharon Davies wrote:

> Dear Professor Waldum,
>
> I sincerely apologise for the continuing delay with publication of your letter.
>
> I am afraid I still cannot give you a publication date as the issue you raise needs to go to our ethics committee, whose next meeting has not been fixed.
>
> Despite the inordinate delay, it is still an important issue. I note also that your letter has not been published on bmj.com. We have an electronic file in our letters database that I could post in response to the article by Dent. Would you like me to do that anyway (even if you decide that you have had enough of waiting and want to withdraw your letter)? If so, I should add something to say that the delay in responding is not yours but mine.
>
> My apologies again for the delay in publishing your letter.
>
> Yours sincerely,
>
> Sharon Davies
> Letters editor

BMJ

2002; 324: 485

Letter:

Helge L. Waldum & Eiliv Brenna.

"Gastro-oesophageal reflux disease in general practice. Last year's guidelines are probably biased"

From the letter:

"Based upon a meeting arranged by the producer of the most used drug in the condition, (AstraZeneca) where the participants were selected by the company and the questions to be raised were formulated in advance, the guidelines for the treatment of gastro-oesophageal reflux disease in general practice were made and later published by authors very close to the company and with the help of said company.

Thus, every step in the process of making the guidelines was controlled by the company."

Over-the-counter PPIs in the US and Norway

Drugs that are used to treat symptoms in prevalent conditions and which have very few, if any, important side effects, may be sold over the counter without a prescription. Before such authorization is granted, there is an evaluation where the risks and benefits are weighed up. In 2000, the FDA arranged such a hearing in Washington, where experts within the field were invited to participate.

I was contacted by the FDA representative I met at the AGA meeting in 1996 and invited to the hearing. I accepted the invitation, stating that I had no connections with the pharmaceutical industry within this field, and that I would be completely competent of making an independent decision. In addition to the FDA staff, four other experts from North America were invited. Considering that the participants should have been completely independent from the pharmaceutical industry, it was a surprise to meet Professor George Sachs there because he has been closely connected to the pharmaceutical companies that produce PPIs since he first described the proton pump (Sachs et al. 1976). He also examined the efficiency of omeprazole (the first PPI produced in Sweden) as an inhibitor of acid secretion).

It was also strange to hear how the other experts were very positive towards the over-the-counter sale of PPIs. Occasionally, they would say something negative, but they would often frame it in the following way: "if I was playing devil's advocate …". I thought that we should show no emotions when discussing the field and, instead, just focus on "pro et contras". In addition to the experts, there were some lay persons at the hearing. During a break, I talked to an old lady, and she asked me why all of the experts had come here to speak for the pharmaceutical industry's interests. Although PPIs apparently have few acute side effects, I tried to focus on problems related to rebound acid hypersecretion, the danger of infections by the oral route in patients lacking gastric acid, and the possible carcinogenic effect of long-term hypergastrinemia. However, there was not much interest in these aspects of the medication.

NTNU
Norwegian University of
Science and Technology

Faculty of Medicine
Department of Intra-Abdominal Diseases

Food and Drug Administration
Center for Drug Evaluation and Research
Division of Gastrointestinal and Coagulation Drug Products, HFD-180
Attn: Document Control Room, Room 6B-24
5600 Fishers Lane
Rockville, MD 20857

Our consultant:

E-mail: berit.myren@medisin.ntnu.no

Dated:	Our ref.:	Your letter dated:	Your ref.:
2001-08-24	2001/HLW/bm	2001-07-10	

Dear Sir,

Enclosed you will find my corrected version from the discussion concerning Prilosec 1. The references are added in the text.

Sincerely yours

Helge L. Waldum
Professor of Medicine

Enclosure

Address	Location	Tel. +47 73 86 85 60	Page 1 of 1
Regionsykehuset i Trondheim	Olav Kyrres g. 17	Fax +47 73 86 75 46	document1
N-7006 Trondheim	Regionsykehuset i Trondheim	Org. no. NO 974 767 880	
Norway			

Page 158

(17) DR. WALDUM: I have a couple of comments (18). First, on pernicious anemia. It is quite clear that there is an increased risk of gastric carcinoma in patients with pernicious anemia (Zamcheck N, Grable E, Ley A, Norman L: Occurrence of gastric cancer among patients with pernicious anemia at the Boston City Hospital. N Engl J Med 1955; 252: 1103-1110, and Elsborg L, Mosbech J. Pernicious anaemia as a risk factor in gastric cancer. Acta Med Scand 1979; 206: 315-318). It is also well documented that patients with pernicious anemia have an increased risk of ECL cell carcinoids (Borch K, Renvall H, Liedberg G. Gastric endocrine cell hyperplasia and carcinoid tumors in patients with pernicious anemia. Gastroenterology 1985; 88: 638-648. Therefore it is difficult for me to understand why you claim that there is no indication for an increased tumor risk in patients with pernicious anemia.

Page 159

Moreover, hypergastrinemia in man results in ECL omas also in Zollinger Ellison syndrome (Bordi G, Cocconi G, Togni R, Vezzadini P, Missale G. Gastric endocrine cell proliferation. Association with Zollinger-Ellison syndrome. Arch Pathol 1974; 98: 274-278). It should be noted that gastrinoma patients not only as a part of multiple endocrine neoplasia, but also the spontaneous type, do develop ECL cell carcinoids (Rindi G, Luinetti O, Cornaggia M, Capella C, Solcia E. Three subtypes of gastric argyrophil carcinoid and he gastric neuroendocrine carcinoma: A clinicopathologic study. Gastroenterology 1993; 104: 994-1006, Cadiot G, Vissuzaine C, Potet F, Mignon M. Fundic argyrophil carcinoid tumor in a patient with sporadic-type Zollinger Ellison syndrome. Dig Dis Sci 1995; 40: 1275-1278).

Therefore, any condition with hypergastrinemia in whatever species, do develop ECL cell carcinoids after prolonged hypergastrinemia (Waldum HL, Petersen H, Brenna E. Gastrin and gastric cancer. Eur J Gastroenterol Hepatol 1992; 4: 801-811). It has been claimed that mice do not develop such tumors, but prolonged treatment with insurmountable histamine 2 antagonist leads to ECL cell carcinoids also in mice (Poynter D, Selway SAM, Papworth SA, Riches SR. Changes in the gastric mucosa of the mouse associated with long lasting unsurmountable histamine H_2 blockade. Gut 1986; 27: 1338-1346). Dosing of omeprazole to dogs for long time, did not result in ECL cell hyperplasia claiming that this species was different from others, and that it did not respond to hypergastrinemia (Säfholm C, Havu N, Forssell H, Sundell G, Mattsson H. Effect of 7 years' daily oral administration of omeprazole to beagle dogs. Digestion 1994; 55: 139-147). However, the dose of omeprazole although comparable to what is dosed in mg/kg for man, did not lead to severe hypoacidity and thus only a modest hypergastrinemia. Therefore it is no reason to claim that the dog is different from other species with respect to trophic effect of gastrin on the ECL cell.

My second comment is related to Helicobacter pylori. Dr. Sachs is apparently unaware of the Norwegian-British study about gastric carcinoma and Helicobacter pylori and gastrin (Hansen S, Vollset SE, Ardill JES, El-Omar E, Melby K, Asse S et al. Hypergastrinaemia is a strong predictor of distal gastric adenocarcinoma among Helicobacter pylori infected persons. Gastroenterology 1997; 112: A575), where the carcinogenic effect of Helicobacter pylori could be completely explained by hypergastrinemia itself. Furthermore, I don't know whether he does know of the American study on transgenic mice being moderately hypergastrinemic, which developed gastric carcinoma (Wang TC, Dangler CA, Chen D, et al. Synergistic interaction between hypergastrinemia and Helicobacter infection in a mouse mode of gastric cancer. Gastroenterology 2000; 118: 36-47), and where Helicobacter pylori-infection augmented the incidence of gastric carcinoma. The additional carcinogenic effect by

2

Helicobacter pylori infection in these moderately hypergastrinemic mice could be explained by the additional hypergastrinemia by Helicobacter pylori-infection (Timothy Wang. Oral presentation. AGA Meeting 2000).

Therefore you have the connection between gastrin and ECL cell tumors in man as well as in animals (Waldum HL, Petersen H, Brenna E. Gastrin and gastric cancer. Eur J Gastroenterol Hepatol 1992; 4: 801-811). It has been claimed that we have not seen any ECL cell tumors in patients treated with omeprazole. However, I should like you to look at page 131 of the sponsors book (Procter Gamble Company/AstraZeneca IP. Omeprazole Magnesium Tablets. Nda no. 21-229, 20 October 2000), where they described 14 cases of gastroduodenal carcinoids and where they could not determine whether the patients had Zollinger Ellison syndrome or pernicious anemia, but also that some of them obviously had acid hypersecretion. I suppose that these patients had gastric acid secretion due to rebound acid hypersecretion, which we described after treatment with omeprazole some years ago (Waldum HL, Arnestad JS, Brenna E, et al. Marked increase in gastric acid secretory capacity after omeprazole treatment. Gut 1996; 39: 649-653), and which later have been confirmed (Gillen D, Wirz A, Ardill JE, et al. Rebound hypersecretion after omeprazole and its relation to on-treatment acid suppression and Helicobacter pylori status. Gastroenterology 1999; 116: 239-247). These 14 patients suggest that ECL cell carcinoids actually develop after treatment with omeprazole. Therefore it would be very interesting to have a completely independent examination of these tumors.

Page 279

(15) DR. WALDUM: I will make a comment regarding H2 blockers and PPI. Although both these types of drugs inhibit gastric acid secretion, there is a great difference between these two groups of patients both regarding efficacy and tolerance. There is a tolerance to H2 blockers (Nwokolo CU, Smith JTL, Gavey C, Sawyer A, Pounder RE. Tolerance during 29 days of conventional dosing with cimetidine, nizatidine, famotidine or ranitidine. Aliment Pharmacol Ther 1990; 4(Suppl. 1): 29-45, Qvigstad G, Arnestad JS, Brenna E, Waldum HL. Treatment with proton pump inhibitors induces tolerance to histamine-2 receptor antagonists in Helicobacter pylori negative patients. Scand J Gastroenterol 1998; 33: 1244-1248), which in the long term reduce the efficacy but also protect them for long-term side effects.

Then I have a comment of the danger of hypergastrinemia. A Finish group published it in the late 80ies (Sjöblom SM, Sipponen P, Karonen SL. Argyrophil cell hyperplasia and carcinoid tumours in oxyntic mucosa of the stomach. Dependence on duration of pernicious anaemia. Eur J gastroenterol hepatol 1991; 3: 153-157) that ECL cell tumors occurred in patients with pernicious anemia, and the incidence of tumors did not increase above gastrin values of 500 pmol. They described tumors also in patients of gastrin values around 100 pmol. They concluded that the risk of ECL cell tumors in hypergastrinemia depended on gastrin values up to a level about 500 pmol and a duration of hypergastrinemia.

I will again underline that ECL cell tumors also occur in mice after prolonged hypergastrinemia (Poynter D, Selway SAM, Papworth SA, Riches SR. Changes in the gastric mucosa of the mouse associated with long lasting unsurmountable histamine H_2 blockade. Gut 1986; 27: 1338-1346). Finally, I will also comment on rebound acid hypersecretion after PPI, which we described as the first group (Waldum HL, Arnestad JS, Brenna E, et al. Marked increase in gastric acid secretory capacity after omeprazole treatment. Gut 1996; 39: 649-653). This gastric acid hypersecretion may be very pronounced reaching values that you otherwise only find in patients with Zollinger Ellison syndrome. Concerning the duration of

3

acid hypersecretion after PPI treatment we have done studies which have not been published yet, showing a duration of the hypersecretion lasting about two – three months with a gradual decline of the hypersecretion during this period.

Although PPIs were not accepted for sale over the counter as a direct result of this meeting, a year later this came to pass. At the hearing, Astra's representatives were present, and I saw the Director of Astra in the US express his thanks to some of the experts for their good performances. I also had a talk with him, and he asked me why I had been invited.

Anyway, the use of PPIs in the US increased further after they were authorized for over-the-counter sale. It is strange that PPIs in fact were granted authorization for over-the-counter sale, including on-demand treatment, since they do not have any immediate symptomatic results, even though the effect on acid secretion persists for hours. Moreover, since there is a considerable variation in their bioavailability and the concentration versus response curve is very steep and shows inter-individual variability in terms of susceptibility, low doses will completely inhibit acid secretion in a few patients but, in others, it will have no effect (Sharma et al. 1984). Thus, even in terms of efficiency, PPIs are not ideal drugs for patient governed use.

Some years later, the Norwegian Medicine Agency had a hearing on whether PPIs should be sold over the counter. I submitted a negative opinion on behalf of our university, but it did not have any impact. Considering that my research group has had an internationally leading position within the research on acid secretion for decades, I have often wondered why. People abroad and at home who claim that I am biased ought to ask themselves why I have taken my job roles. I could have had a much better life being a part of the mainstream and cooperating with the pharmaceutical industry. However, my standards are based upon studies which nobody has disproved. To seek the truth has always been my guiding star. After PPIs were accepted over-the-counter in Norway, I wrote a letter presenting my arguments against this move (H. L. Waldum 2009). Others stated that PPIs did not cause cancer (Hatlebakk, Lerang, and Moum 2010) and I responded to their arguments (H. L. Waldum 2010).

Tidsskriftet
-Den norske Legeforening-
(H.L. Waldum 2010)

Proton pump inhibitors over-the-counter

"I read with some surprise the somewhat emotional correspondence [Hatlebakk, Lerang, and Moum, 2010] on my letter on proton pump inhibitors sold over-the-counter [Waldum HL 2009].

It seemed that the authors were not familiar with the Danish study where healthy students were given proton pump inhibitors for a period and, some days after stopping the drug, developed dyspepsia [Reimer, Sondergaard, Hilsted, et al. 2009] probably due to rebound acid hypersecretion [Waldum, Arnestad, Brenna 1996].

They claimed that the clinical relevance of rebound acid hypersecretion after proton pump inhibitors has not been shown. Why should rebound acid hypersecretion not aggravate gastro-esophageal reflux disease, when it causes such symptoms in healthy individuals?

An important principle was not followed when a compound that creates malignant tumors in its target organ was accepted for clinical use.

In meetings arranged by Astra around 1990 where pathologists and gastroenterologists agreed that omeprazole was safe in the short and long-term despite the tumors induced in rats. I would add that it would have been appropriate if the journal had asked the authors (Hatlebakk, Lerang, Moum,2010) of the letter about financial support from the pharmaceutical industry.

Finally, I will express that I agree that atrophic gastritis gives higher gastrin values than treatment with proton pump inhibitors. But do they not know that atrophic gastritis is the most important factor in gastric carcinogenesis? I will repeat my statement that those who believe more in studies over a limited time period than evolution lack biological knowledge."

Evaluations at the Norwegian Research Council

During the last two decades, it has become customary to have international evaluations of our research in Norway. Two such evaluations have been performed in the name of the Norwegian Research Council. The purpose of these evaluations is to have a great impact on scientific funding. Indeed, the evaluation grades have significant implications for research funding.

I had great expectations for the first of these evaluations, hoping that the committee would be able to see beyond the journals publishing the research, and instead focus on who had published important new findings first. During the last 25 years, we have been at the forefront of research: our description of the regulation of histamine release from the ECL cell (Sandvik et al. 1987; Brenna and Waldum 1991); the localization of the gastrin receptor (Bakke et al. 2001); the concentration dependency of the trophic effect of gastrin on the ECL cell, which reaches a maximum at a much lower gastrin concentration than anticipated (Brenna and Waldum 1992); the important role of the ECL cell in human carcinogenesis (H. L. Waldum et al. 1991; H. L. Waldum et al. 1998; Qvigstad et al. 1999; Qvigstad et al. 2000; Qvigstad et al. 2002; H. L. Waldum and Brenna 1993); and contributions to a new classification of human gastric carcinomas (H. L. Waldum and Brenna 1993). Moreover, we were the first to publish the correct location of the gastrin receptor (Bakke et al. 2001) and the rebound acid hypersecretion caused by PPIs (H. L. Waldum et al. 1996). Both these findings were quoted on the front page of *Gastroenterology* but from other people's research which took place after ours, and we were not given any credit. However, I was very disappointed with the evaluation, which was probably a bit naive given the number of Swedes on the committee who had a relationship with Astra.

During the interview, I immediately sensed hostility from some members of the committee. For instance, we were attacked for struggling to achieve funding for our research. As I see it, producing a lot of research without spending a lot of money should be seen as a good thing and not a bad one. We also discussed the relationship to the pharmaceutical industry, and a Danish member of the committee asked why we did not cooperate with them. This told me that this expert was either connected to the pharmaceutical industry or, if not, that he was very naïve.

Along with this bad rating, we were advised to cooperate with other units at our hospital/university. It is difficult to see how this would have improved our research, since the proposed units were not at our scientific level. After receiving the low rating, I started to look more closely at the competence of the members of the committee and found that one of the Swedes had a connection to Astra. As often is the case in such situations, the organization arranging the evaluation stands by the committee members against the few that are appealing. Those appealing are à priori considered to be bad losers. Given that this bad rating was an important evaluation, I realized that I would have problems getting money for our research at the national level. I still received money from local sources, which made it possible to continue my work, although I always had to use as little money as possible. Over time, however, local funding in Trondheim became increasingly concentrated on a few people based upon a defined strategy.

It is a sad fact that our work has never been given any priority, although we started doing translational research at least ten years before anyone else. Moreover, our collection of blood and tissue from patients with gastric cancer started about ten years before biobanks became popular. Furthermore, my group has produced most theses in our hospital and our candidates have all excelled. I have never understood why we have received such limited local funding in the last decade. Is it due to my open criticisms of people in leading positions, or does the pharmaceutical companies' influence even reach here?

NTNU
Norwegian University of Science and Technology

Faculty of Medicine
Department of Cancer Research and Molecular Medicine

Norwegian Research Council

Dated:	Our ref.:	Your letter dated:	Your ref.:
2004-11-12			

The evaluation of clinical research 2003
A question of competence of the committee and particularly the secretary Henrik Sjövall

Norwegian Research Council organized last year an evaluation of clinical research in Norway. I looked forward to this and also participated in the oral presentation. At that presentation I immediately notised the unfriendly atmosphere. Thus, it was concentrated on my low funding resources. No attempt to assess my research in connection with my funding (in other words my efficiency) was done. Moreover, I was asked about my negative writing concerning drug induced hypoacidity and was directly asked why I did no co-operate with pharmaceutical industry, and in this context it means Astra Zeneca. I felt during this oral presentation before the Evaluation Committee that non-scientific interests were involved. At the end of the day I raised a question about possible relationship between members of the committee and pharmaceutical industry, particularly Astra Zeneca. The reason was that I have worked for nearly 30 years with gastrin and during the last 20 years produced results and scientific publications focusing on the negative aspects of profound acid inhibition. Thus I had perpetually given evidence for risk of human gastric carcinomas during prolonged acid inhibition and even published a paper indicating that inhibition of acid secretion would make persons more susceptible to prion diseases, including new variant Creutzfelt Jakob disease.

Taking into consideration that omeprazole/esomeprazole from Astra Zeneca is world-wide the most sold drug, my research may have negative impact on that company. I will therefore claim that anybody having any close connection with Astra Zeneca will be disqualified to give a fair evaluation of my research. A negative evaluation was indeed made. Thus, when comparing my publications both in number and in impact factor of the journals, there are little if any differences between groups that got two degrees higher rating. Moreover, my group had produced most theses by medical doctors. This was mentioned but apparently did not have any influence on the final rating. It is also strange that the fact that our results and findings have implications for other organ systems was said to be a negative factor and not a positive one. It was claimed that our research was too less focused. This is very unfair and I enclose the overview of the title of the theses produced by our group, showing that gastrin and gastric acidity and neuroendocrinology are common subjects in all these theses. At the oral presentation I therefore protested against the Chairman, Professor Ulf Smith, claiming that our research was not focused.

The committee was very dominated by Swedes and even Swedes from Gothenburg. Knowing the influence Astra Zeneca has on Swedish research and particularly in the Gothenburg area, I

Address
St. Olavs Hospital HF
NO-7006 Trondheim
ikm-post@medisin.ntnu.no

Location
Kreftbygget
Olav Kyrres gt 17
www.medisin.ntnu.no/ikm

Tel. +47 73 86 72 71
Fax +47 73 86 72 89
Org. no. NO 974 767 880

immediately suspected non-scientific influence on the evaluation of my research. When returning from the oral evaluation in Oslo I therefore looked for Astra Zeneca connection between the participants in the committee, but could not find direct proof for it. Later I become aware of Henrik Sjövall as being the secretary of the committee. He has a long co-operation with people closely connected to Astra Zeneca and I will claim that he is ineligible in evaluation my research. Since the secretary naturally has great influence on the written report I will accordingly claim that the evaluation of my research was made by a committee that was ineligible. Since this evaluation report has been spread throughout the country and will have influence of the allocation of resources for many years to come, I will accordingly ask for a new evaluation by a committee not influenced by Astra Zeneca or any other relevant firm.

I have not much hope for any positive change in the evaluation of our research. Nevertheless, I find it of importance to have this letter sent so that the Norwegian Research Council cannot claim that they were not aware of commercial influence on the evaluation. Potent gastric acid inhibition has recently been reported to increase the risk of pneumonia, and proximal gastric cancers and particularly those of diffuse type are increasing in frequency supporting that our results and our research for fifteen years may soon be generally accepted. In the context of the recent scandal with Vioxx, it should be obvious even to the Norwegian Research Council that the interest of the community and science is not the same as that of pharmaceutical companies.

Sincerely yours

Helge L. Waldum
Professor of Medicine

Page 2 of 2
nfr evaluering av forskningen, nov04.doc

1.3. Committee Evaluation:

1.3.1. Scientific output: [redacted]

1.3.2. Leadership: [redacted]

1.3.3. General comments: [redacted]

2. Institute of Cancer and Molecular Medicine

2.1. Department structure and funding situation: [redacted]

2.2. Summary of SWOT analysis: This analysis was not done at the institute level, as intended, but at the unit level. It was, therefore, available only for the most scientifically active sections. The GI unit has a positive outlook, with good recruitment of PhD's, including those with a medical background. Access to equipment is not considered to be a problem. The unit seems to be steering in the direction of general oncology. [redacted]

2.2 Summary of SWOT analysis: This analysis was not done at the institute level, as intended, but at the unit level. It was, therefore, available only for the most scientifically active sections The GI unit has a positive outlook, with good recruitment of PhD's, including those with a medical background. Access to equipment is not considered to be a problem. The unit seems to be steering in the direction of general oncology.

51

. **Committee Evaluation:**

2.3.1. Scientific output: Fair to excellent

2.3.2. Leadership:

2.3.3. General comments:

The GI group has a good scientific output but seems isolated. It is currently moving in the direction of general oncology rather than focusing on GI issues. It is the opinion of the Committee that the unit would benefit from more cooperation with other GI groups, both internally and externally. One way to accomplish this would be to create a Center for Digestive Diseases. We also note that the Institute for Circulation and Medical imaging has a very high competence in medical technology that might be used to enlarge the technical platform of the GI unit. The prospect of an entirely new building also raises the possibility of trying to build up an "Operating room of the future" with a GI profile. This opportunity, if marketed correctly, should make it possible to recruit new clinical scientists to the unit, provided that the current leaders are willing to take on this challenge. The need to establish a multidisciplinary digestive disease group is a crucial task for the institution to again become internationally competitive.

Application for a professorship in Stockholm

After I left Tromsø in 1981 and moved to Trondheim, which is close to my birthplace, I applied for two professorships in Oslo and Stockholm.

In the Oslo evaluation, I was given the highest rating among the gastroenterologists, but two people from other subspecialties were given higher ratings overall. At 60 years old, I applied for a position at Karolinska Hospital, Stockholm. The original committee consisted of Professor Jenny Heathcote, Toronto; Professor Jan Tack, Leuven; and Professor Åke Nilsson, Lund. They gave separate statements and obviously could not reach an agreement. In my opinion, only Professor Åke Nilsson evaluated me fairly. Professor Heathcote gave me the lowest possible score in science, teaching, clinical skills, leadership, development, and collaboration; my total rating was far below the others. Professor Jan Tack rated me the lowest in nearly all aspects.

Since the committee was not able to give a common statement, Professor Erik Schrumpf, Oslo, was asked to make a new evaluation. He gave a thorough and fair evaluation, and awarded me second place. In retrospect, it is difficult to understand how and why Professor Heathcote and Professor Tack could give such low ratings based upon the available data.

Meeting at the International Agency for Research on Cancer (IARC) and the World Health organization (WHO), Lyon, December 1999

I was invited to participate in a meeting on the "Predictive value of rodent forestomach gastric neuroendocrine tumors in evaluating carcinogenic risks in humans."

I was very pleased with the subject and for being invited to the meeting. My university colleague, Professor Duan Chen, was also invited, and so Trondheim was well represented at this meeting. I felt that there would finally be a meeting without commercial influence arranged by an international organization that demonstrated its independence and neutrality by inviting us. Moreover, the other participants were not among those I considered too closely connected to the pharmaceutical industry. The meeting was interesting, and we had very good discussions. At the close of the meeting we were asked to submit a manuscript from our presentation, which would be included in a book of the proceedings. The organizer stated that they wanted to finish this book within a few months.

I think all the participants completed their manuscript within the scheduled time. However, the book did not appear. After more than six months, I started to write letters asking when it would be published. After some time, the organizer replied that the book had been delayed because some of the people involved in the process had left their positions. Therefore, they did not have enough people to do the work. I continued to ask for the book at monthly intervals. After about two years, I was told that the book would appear sooner if I stopped asking and allowed them to do the work rather than spending time answering my letters.

After 30 months, I realized that the book would never be published, unless I acted. At that time the former prime minister of Norway and MD, Gro Harlem Brundtland, was the leader of WHO. I, therefore, wrote a letter to her, indicating that commercial interests were trying to stop the book. Shortly afterwards, it was published with our contribution(H. L Waldum, Qvigstad, and Brenna 2003). It is difficult to avoid the impression that some external forces were attempting to stop or delay the book resulting from this meeting.

WORLD HEALTH ORGANIZATION

ORGANISATION MONDIALE DE LA SANTE

CENTRE INTERNATIONAL DE RECHERCHE SUR LE CANCER
INTERNATIONAL AGENCY FOR RESEARCH ON CANCER

150, COURS ALBERT-THOMAS, 69372 LYON CEDEX 08, FRANCE

Tél. 04 72 73 84 85 Télex 380 023 Télécopie 04 72 73 85 75 & 04 72 73 83 19
International tel: +33 472 73 84 85; direct tel: +33 472 73 84 76
International fax: +33 472 73 85 75; direct fax: +33 472 73 83 19
e-mail: rice@iarc.fr

IARC FACSIMILE

From: Dr J.M. Rice

To: Prof. Helge L. Waldum

Ref.

Fax No. +47 73 86 ~~85 60~~ 75-46

Date: 1 July 2000

Page 1 of 1 page

Dear Professor Waldum,

The editing of the proceedings of the symposium on Predictive Value of Forestomach and Gastric Neuroendocrine Tumours in Rodents in Carcinogenic Hazard Identification is well advanced, and you should receive your edited contribution during the first half of July.

The book should be printed this autumn.

Yours sincerely,

Jerry M. Rice

Jerry M. Rice, Ph.D.
Chief,
Unit of Carcinogen Identification
and Evaluation

NTNU
Norwegian University of
Science and Technology

Faculty of Medicine
Department of Intra-Abdominal Diseases

Fax

To:	Jerry M. Rice	Fax:	33 472 73 85 75
From:	Helge L. Waldum	Fax:	+47 73 86 75 46

No. of pages incl. this:
In case you do not receive all pages, please call: +47 73 86 85 41

Date: 2001-03-30

Message:

Dear Jerry M. Rice,

I appreciated the possibility to read the proof of my contribution to the book concerning the Safety of proton pump inhibitors and the relevance of animal studies.

Do you have any information of when the book will arrive? The reason why asking, is that I get many questions regarding this book.

Sincerely yours

Helge L. Waldum
Professor of Medicine

Address
Regionsykehuset i Trondheim
N-7006 Trondheim
Norway

Location
Olav Kyrres g. 17
Regionsykehuset i Trondheim

Tel. +47 73 86 85 60
Fax +47 73 86 75 46

Page 1 of 1
document3

file:///U

OK? 17 sendt

Dear Dr. Rice,

I am again asking you about the book related to the IARC Gastric Tumour Meeting in November 1999. The last time i heard from you was in December 2000, and it was then promised that the book would appear early in 2001. Since I still have not got any new information, and many people are asking me what is going on, I contact you again to know when the book will appear.

Sincerely yours
Helge L. Waldum
Professor of Medicine

WORLD HEALTH ORGANIZATION

ORGANISATION MONDIALE DE LA SANTE

INTERNATIONAL AGENCY FOR RESEARCH ON CANCER
CENTRE INTERNATIONAL DE RECHERCHE SUR LE CANCER

150, cours Albert Thomas 69008 Lyon France http://www.iarc.fr/

To all participants in the
Workshop on Predictive Value of Gastric Neuroendocrine and Forestomach Tumours in Rodents for Carcinogenic Hazard Identification, Lyon, 29.11.99-01.12.99

Unit of Carcinogen Identification and Evaluation
Tel. : +33 4 72 73 84 76
Fax : +33 4 72 73 83 19
E-mail: cie@iarc.fr

http://monographs.iarc.fr

Ref.: Status of the Proceedings

21 February 2002

Dear Participant,

This is to inform you of the current status of the Proceedings of the above-referenced Workshop, the publication of which has been delayed by circumstances beyond our control.

Briefly, IARC offered early retirement to all its long-serving regular-budget employees during the autumn of 2000, to compensate for a budgetary shortfall that had resulted from two member states (Argentina and Brazil) having left the Agency. Three of the ten staff members of this Unit accepted this offer, and all retired in December 2000. Since then it has been necessary to prioritize our activities very strictly in order to maintain the key elements of our programme, of which the *Monographs* themselves have highest priority.

Mr Julian Wilbourn, who was working on the Proceedings document, was one of those who elected to retire. At the time he left, the document was in an advanced state but was still incomplete. Julian's vacant position and one other position in this Unit were subsequently abolished by decision of the IARC Director. Since then we have found ourselves extremely understaffed.

Since Julian's departure I have taken on the task of completing the Proceedings myself, in such time as I can take from other responsibilities. The current status is the following:

- The revised and edited papers of individual authors have been prepared for the printer in Quark format; only a final proofreading is required.
- Excellent colour photomicrographs for the cover of the book have been furnished by Dr Ron Herbert, illustrating both kinds of neoplasm at low and high magnifications.
- The editing of the consensus statements for both kinds of tumour is all that remains to be completed. The statement for forestomach tumours, however, is in the form of a rough draft and needs significant additional attention.

02 02 11:06 FAX 0472738318 CIE 003

21 Feb. 2002

2

I expect that the final text will be completed this spring and that you will receive your copies of the printed book by summer. I regret that it has taken so long to complete the work, but I must ask for your continued patience for a few more months in order that we may ultimately have a volume of which we can all be proud.

Thank you for your continuing interest in the Proceedings of this meeting.

Yours sincerely,

Jerry M. Rice, PhD
Chief, Unit of Carcinogen
Identification and Evaluation

NTNU
Norwegian University of Science and Technology

Faculty of Medicine
Department of Intra-Abdominal Diseases

Dr. Gro Harlem Bruntland
Director-General
World Health Organization
Avenue Appia 20
1211 Geneva 27
Switzerland

Telephone no.:

Dated:	Our ref.:	Your letter dated:	Your ref.:
2002-10-14	2002/HLW/bm		

Dear Gro Harlem Bruntland,

Late in 1998 I among about 15 researchers was invited by International Agency for Research on Cancer (IARC), World Health Organization (WHO), to participate in a meeting in November 1999 on the relevance of rodent studies concerning development of gastric tumours after long-term acid inhibition with respect to man. I was delighted about this since I for a long time had fronted this issue internationally against pharmaceutical industry and scientists more or less connected to pharmaceutical companies. The meeting was interesting and open, and it was stressed that we had to deliver the manuscript at the meeting or immediately afterwards, in order to publish the book from the meeting within six months, which was the standard policy of IARC.

Now, nearly three years afterwards, no book has appeared, and I enclose proof of my contribution and some of the correspondence I have had with IARC about the issue. I am sorry to put on paper that I cannot avoid the thought that pharmaceutical industry could have interfered with the publishing process. Each year they can postpone the appearance of the book could mean a lot for them economically, and be potentially harmful for the patients.

For your information I enclose some relevant publications that I have written about the issue.

Please give an answer to this letter.

Sincerely yours

Helge L. Waldum
Professor of Medicine

Copy: Chief Jerry M. Rice, IARC, Unit of Carcinogen

Enclosure

Address	Location			
St. Olavs Hospital HF	Olav Kyrres g. 17	Tel.	+47 73 86 85 60	Page 1 of 1
N-7006 Trondheim	St. Olavs Hospital HF	Fax	+47 73 86 75 46	11
Norway		Org. no.	NO 974 767 880	

Hypergastrinemia and gastric cancer in humans

With the development and use of radioimmunoassay, which determines gastrin in the blood, it became evident that long-term hypergastrinemia in humans resulted in the development of ECL cell derived gastric carcinoids, whether the hypergastrinemia was secondary to reduced gastric acid secretion (Sjoblom et al. 1989) or due to a gastrin-producing tumor inducing increased gastric acid secretion (Solcia et al. 1990).

Thus, in the eighties, an Italian specialist in pathology, Bordi, wrote an article on ECL cell carcinoids as a hormone-induced tumor (Bordi 1988). With the description of the rats' malignant tumors, which had been induced by long-term omeprazole dosing (Havu 1986), the focus had apparently shifted away from the role of gastrin in human tumorigenesis. Although, that said, it was also recognized that the tumors in the rats were ECL cell derived, secondary to hypergastrinemia, which was due to drug induced hypoacidity.

It was claimed that the rat was special, and that the ECL cell derived tumors in humans were not due to hypergastrinemia alone, as they occurred in patients with atrophic gastritis. This means that they believed that they primarily resulted from inflammation and the condition was only partially due to hypergastrinemia. Similarly, ECL cell carcinoids in patients with gastrinoma only occurred in people with multiple endocrine neoplasia type I (MEN I), where there was a genetic error predisposing them to neuroendocrine tumors (Berna et al. 2008). Another Italian specialist in the area put this into a system (Rindi et al. 1993) that classified ECL cell carcinoids, according to their cause: type 1 secondary to atrophic gastritis, type 2 secondary to gastrinoma as part of MEN I, and type 3 without hypergastrinemia. However, even at the time, it was known that some patients with gastrinoma without MEN I could develop ECL cell carcinoids (Cadiot et al. 1995; Feurle 1994), thereby showing that hypergastrinemia alone was enough to cause this type of tumor. It must, however, be admitted that there is a higher frequency of ECL cell carcinoids in gastrinoma patients as part of MEN I, than in those without this genetic abnormality. However, it is clinically true that gastrinomas in patients with MEN I are more benign than those occurring in persons without it. Moreover, in contrast to gastrinomas occurring in patients with MEN I, which are often multiple, those developing in patients without MEN I are more often solitary, and therefore amenable to surgery. Patients with gastrinomas as part of MEN I often live longer with hypergastrinemia than those with gastrinomas without an apparent cause. This means that tumors from the slow proliferating ECL cell will have a longer time to develop in MEN I patients.

Furthermore, with regard to the rat's specific susceptibility to ECL tumor development, Astra completed studies on dogs and mice instead, where no such tendency was found, even at a rather high dose (Safholm et al. 1994; Ekman et al. 1985). In mice, PPIs were not prone to inducing ECL cell derived tumors unlike an insurmountable histamine-2 blocker (Poynter et al. 1986). However, PPIs only induce ECL cell derived tumors when they cause marked hypoacidity and secondary hypergastrinemia. Accordingly, dog and particularly mice (Martinsen et al. 2011), are very resistant to the acid inhibitory effect of PPIs. In these dog and mouse studies, PPIs were not dosed sufficiently high enough to induce the biological effect of inhibiting gastric acidity, which is sought in therapy. Accordingly, they are not of any value when assessing the long-term safety of PPI treatments in humans. However, histamine-2 blockers, like the insurmountable loxtidine, are efficient inhibitors of acid secretion in mice, and they also induce ECL cell derived tumors in that species [Poynter et al. 1986]. Considering the many hundreds of reviews and articles written on PPI use and safety, it is curious that these aspects have only been discussed by our group. At a large meeting in Monte Carlo in November 1988, Astra (L. Sölvel) concluded that "All experience with omeprazole to date indicates it to be safe without any specific side-effect pattern." Accordingly, animal studies were not included in the safety evaluation.

Experience with journals and conferences

When I started within research, I thought that new important findings would be welcomed immediately, so long as the applied methods were adequate and properly performed. During my career, however, I have learned that this is not the case. The most popular manuscripts are those supporting the views of a previous study, particularly if that study has been done by an influential person within the field. Moreover, when our group has completed studies which have results that do not agree with the prevailing theory, we have always tried to find the reason for the discrepancy. When doing so, we have always first carefully examined our own study for errors and biases. If we cannot find any faults there, then we will look for errors in studies with conflicting results by others. Looking for mistakes in other people's studies is not a popular act but, in my opinion, it is necessary in scientific practice.

When we were the first group to begin to do histamine determination using the commercially available radioimmunoassay method, our work was evaluated by to W. Lorenz, who had dominated histamine determination for at least a decade using a chemical method (Lorenz et al. 1991). Although his chemical method was intrinsically less sensitive than a radioimmunoassay, he managed to stop our paper from being published in *Gut* by stating that, in his method, many hundred compounds had been shown not to interfere with the assay, whereas only a few had been tested using the radioimmunoassay method. However, due to the inherent specificity of a radioimmunoassay, it is acceptable to only test closely related substances. Of course, only a short time after we first used the radioimmunoassay method for histamine determination, everybody started to adopt it because of its sensitivity and specificity. Interestingly, we found that the trophic effect of gastrin on the ECL cell in rats showed the same concentration dependency as the functional effect [Brenna and Waldum 1992]: that is, stimulating the release of histamine.

We submitted the manuscript to *Gastroenterology* and it was returned, requesting minor changes, which normally indicates that it would be accepted for publication. However, in the meantime, *Gastroenterology* had a change of editor, who rejected the manuscript. It is difficult to avoid assuming that it was rejected because it showed that maximal functional and trophic effects were reached at a lower gastrin concentration than previously realized, and that Sjøblom et al. had previously shown that the maximal trophic effect of gastrin in patients with pernicious anemia occurred at the same level (Sjoblom et al. 1989).

Altogether, these findings suggested that even moderately elevated gastrin concentrations in many patients treated with proton pump inhibitors could induce ECL cell neoplasia. This experience made me realize that I would never get any manuscripts accepted by *Gastroenterology*, and I did not submit any more manuscripts to this journal. For a while, however, they accepted my letters which indicated errors and problems in published papers, and I profited from this opportunity before it was shut down. I have already described my experience with *The Lancet*, that would not accept our manuscript showing that rebound acid hypersecretion probably leads to physical dependency after treatment with omeprazole, which was the most sold drug at the time. I have also mentioned the problems having a letter about the obviously biased guidelines for the treatment of reflux esophagitis published in the *BMJ*. Although there was also a period where I had problems getting manuscripts accepted in *GUT*, this journal has been fairer when evaluating our manuscripts. I am also very pleased that the *Scandinavian Journal of Gastroenterology* has published most of our work. I am presently the Editor-in-Chief of this journal which, throughout its 50-

year history, has been completely independent and free of commercial influence.

During the last twenty-five years, my main interest has been within pathology, especially gastric cancer. It has always been hard to get our manuscripts accepted, as their results and interpretations were at odds with existing beliefs. Although our findings indirectly incriminated hypergastrinemia, and therefore the use of inhibitors of gastric acid secretion, in the tumorigenic process, my impression has been that the negativity towards our work in pathology journals has been based on a reluctance to accept new ideas, rather than on connections to the pharmaceutical industry. From a scientific view, it is not acceptable to refuse a manuscript because you dislike its results, even though it is not possible to find methodological weaknesses to explain the diverging conclusions. The subjectivity of manuscript evaluation was amply demonstrated when one of our most important manuscripts, which showed that there was no mucin gene expression in gastric cancer cells of the signet ring cell type, was refused by four journals of pathology, but accepted directly by the editor of the fifth journal (Sørdal et al. 2014). This journal has an impact factor above most of the journals which had rejected the article.

Another way to suppress the importance, and thus the impact, of a scientist is to never refer to papers written by them. Although we have been the first group to describe many findings, we have not been cited. The best example is our work on rebound acid hypersecretion, which the McColl group copied and then published on it more than two years later [Gillen et al. 1999]. Nevertheless, many authors have consequently referred to McColl's and omitted to mention ours. Also, our work is seldom referred to within pathology, despite the fact that we have published in this field since 1990. However, strangely, nobody has disapproved our results.

Another area where economic interests are involved is conferences. I have attended the yearly "Digestive Disease Week (DDW)" about 35 times, and I was initially disappointed when my submitted abstracts were not accepted for oral presentation. After some time, I realized that I would not be allowed to speak at this meeting, and the best I could achieve was to have a poster on the last day. Looking at the pharmaceutical company names on the material distributed to the delegates, it became evident that the PPI producers, particularly AstraZeneca, were the sponsors, and, therefore, it would be naïve to believe that they did not have an influence over the scientific program.

I hope that it has also become evident to my readers that publishing scientific results that have negative consequences for the pharmaceutical companies is often difficult. This is particularly true for results that indicate long-term side effects, such as cancer. It should be realized that cancer development is often is a slow process, which is demonstrated by the fact that it most often occurs in the elderly.

Gastroenterology
March 1996 Volume 110
Number 3

Front Cover:

Figure depicting that gastrin stimulates gastric acid secretion solely by stimulating histamine release from the ECL cell without having any effect on the parietal cell.

A letter from us related to this figure:

Helge L. Waldum, Arne K. Sandvik, Eiliv Brenna, Per M. Kleveland.
The Gastrin-Histamine Sequence. *Gastroenterology* 1996 (3);
volume 111: 838-839.

"It was fascinating to find a figure on the front page showing that gastrin stimulated acid secretion by solely interacting with the ECL cell, but sad to see that we were not referred to, although we had already published this figure in 1991 and in other later publications with some small modifications."

Letter to the Food and Drug Administration (FDA) and "Public Citizen", Washington

Some years ago, I was contacted by Director Sidney Wolfe from "Public Citizen" about the safety of PPIs. Together, we prepared a 39-page document describing our concerns, where Wolfe expressed fears over the increased risk of fractures and infections, whereas I focused on rebound acid hypersecretion, physical dependency, and the risk of neoplasia.

We asked for boxed warnings. Our letter was commented on in *GI & Hepatology News* (2011, 5: 16–18) by Professor Metz, who was interviewed, along with six other experts. Interestingly, all of these experts denied any neoplastic risk related to PPIs; they also minimized the problem of rebound acid hypersecretion, which was a phenomenon that some of them doubted existed.

It is sad to see that so-called experts can deny the existence of rebound acid hypersecretion by referring to studies with a design that could not have disclosed this phenomenon. Perhaps, these studies were performed to confuse readers; otherwise they must have been designed by researchers without any knowledge of gastric physiology.

With regard to the neoplastic effect of hypergastrinemia, which is secondary to the inhibition of acid secretion, some of the "experts" claim that the results in rats are peculiar and that two decades of use shows that there is no risk. However, are these "experts" not aware of the fact that, when long-term safety is being evaluated, small animals are used because all the processes move faster in them? One year for a rat is comparable to 25 to 30 years in humans.

Cancer is a disease that takes time to develop and is, therefore, mainly a disease of the elderly. This means that we must rely on animal studies when assessing the risk of neoplasia. This principle was not followed when the first PPI was authorized for clinical use. Interestingly, many of the "experts" have a history of close connections to the PPI producers.

PUBLICCITIZEN

NEWS RELEASE

1600 20th Street, NW • Washington, D.C. 20009 • 202/588-1000 • www.citizen.org

EMBARGOED UNTIL:
10 a.m. EDT Aug. 23, 2011

Contact: Angela Bradbery (202) 588-7741
Dorry Samuels (202) 588-7742

Many Popular Stomach Acid-Reducing Drugs Are Habit-Forming, Dangerous

Nexium, Prilosec and Other Proton Pump Inhibitors Are Overprescribed, Should Carry Strongest Possible Warning, Public Citizen Tells FDA in Petition

WASHINGTON, D.C. – Many widely prescribed stomach acid-reducing drugs can cause long-term dependence and should carry the strongest possible warning label for this and several other dangerous adverse effects, Public Citizen told the U.S. Food and Drug Administration (FDA) in a petition sent today.

The drugs are proton pump inhibitors (PPIs), so-named because of the mechanism they use to shut off the production of stomach acid. PPIs are one of the most widely used classes of drugs in the United States, with 119 million prescriptions dispensed in 2009 and $13.6 billion in U.S. sales. An estimated 1 of every 20 people in the developed world is taking the medications, which include Nexium, Dexilant, Prilosec, Prilosec OTC, Zegerid, Zegerid OTC, Prevacid, Prevacid 24-Hr, Protonix, Aciphex, Vimovo and numerous generic counterparts, most prominently omeprazole and pantoprazole.

"These drugs are being prescribed far too commonly to people who shouldn't be taking them," said Dr. Sidney Wolfe, director of Public Citizen's Health Research Group. "As a result, millions of people are needlessly setting themselves up to become dependent on PPIs while exposing themselves to the serious risks associated with long-term therapy. The FDA should act immediately to ensure that patients and physicians are adequately warned of these effects, and reminded of the many safer alternatives for common conditions such as acid reflux."

PPIs are approved to treat gastroesophageal reflux disease (GERD) – sometimes referred to as acid reflux – as well as gastric ulcers, erosive esophagitis and stomach bleeding associated with using non-steroidal anti-inflammatory drugs (NSAIDs). But evidence shows that after using

PPIs for a month or more, patients who stop taking the drug make even more stomach acid than before they started the drug, a phenomenon known as rebound acid hypersecretion, which causes acid reflux symptoms to return even worse than before therapy. The symptoms prompt patients to begin taking the PPI again, creating a long-term dependence on these drugs, particularly worrisome for the large number of patients who did not even need the drugs in the first place. As Dr. K.E. McColl, a leading Scottish researcher on adverse effects of PPI use, recently concluded, "The current finding that these drugs induce symptoms [after withdrawal] means that such liberal [mis-] prescribing is likely to be creating the disease the drugs are designed to treat and causing patients with no previous need for such therapy to require intermittent or long-term treatment."

In addition to creating dependency, PPIs increase the risk for several serious conditions, including fractures of the hip, spine and wrist; an increased risk of serious infections such as pneumonia and *C. difficile* diarrhea; and severe magnesium deficiency, which can cause life-threatening cardiac arrhythmias. PPIs also may reduce the effectiveness of other drugs used to treat heart attacks and cancer, and in some cases, can cause vitamin B12 deficiency and kidney failure. Although some of these side effects already are mentioned somewhere in the labels (not the case for the dependence), none – including those that are life-threatening – are displayed prominently as black box warnings, the strongest possible warning.

Therefore, physicians may not be aware of the serious risks associated with PPI therapy, resulting in a large number of unnecessary prescriptions. Studies have shown that up to two-thirds of all people taking PPIs do not even have a condition that the drugs are designed to treat, and the drugs are often taken for much longer periods of time than they are approved for. In addition, PPIs are commonly prescribed for conditions such as acid reflux that could be treated with safer alternatives that are often just as effective.

Public Citizen is petitioning the FDA to require that more prominent black box warnings and other safety information be added to the product labels of all PPIs on the market. Public Citizen also is calling for patient medication guides to be distributed with all PPIs and for the makers of the drugs to send a letter to doctors alerting them to these adverse effects and of the need to try safer alternatives first for conditions such as GERD.

Dr. Helge L. Waldum, a co-petitioner with Public Citizen, is head of the Department of Digestive and Liver Diseases at Trondheim University Hospital in Norway and author of 135 medical journal articles related to the topics of this petition, among them the first trial to show that patients could become dependent on PPIs through the rebound effect. In a statement released today, he noted: "Given that most people on PPIs long-term may not even have a documented need for the medication, and that for those that are on these drugs for legitimate reasons, several safer alternatives exist, the risks greatly outweigh any benefit in most patients on PPIs. I therefore urge the FDA to act promptly on the recommendations outlined in this petition."

Robert Kuttner, a well-known journalist and co-editor of the *American Prospect*, long suffered from severe acid reflux and became dependent on PPIs after a particularly severe episode. After years of unsuccessfully trying to control his symptoms with ever higher doses of the PPI, the reflux resolved only after a physician tapered him off the drug to another therapy. Now largely symptom-free, Kuttner, who released a statement today in support of Public Citizen's petition, concluded: "My experience certainly seems to confirm the pattern of PPI medication causing – or in my case, seriously aggravating – the condition that it supposedly treats. In my case, the PPI seemed to have primed my system to produce increasing amounts of acid so that over time I was more prone to more attacks triggered by ever more minor departures from a very low fat diet … The ever-increasing amounts of PPI helped only temporarily and required dependence on even higher doses, and so on, over several cycles. Only getting off the PPI reversed what seemed to be a chronic and progressive condition."

To read the petition, visit: http://www.citizen.org/documents/1964.pdf.

To read Dr. Helge Waldum's statement of support, visit http://www.citizen.org/documents/Waldum_statement_in_support_of_HRG_petition.pdf.

To read Robert Kuttner's full statement in support of the petition, visit http://www.citizen.org/documents/Kuttner_statement_in_support_of_HRG_petition.pdf.

###

Public Citizen is a national, nonprofit consumer advocacy organization based in Washington, D.C. For more information, please visit www.citizen.org.

[Date Sent]

Margaret A. Hamburg, M.D.
Commissioner
U.S. Food and Drug Administration
Department of Health and Human Services
WO 2200
10903 New Hampshire Avenue
Silver Spring, MD 20993-0002

Dear Dr. Hamburg,

As a physician and life-long researcher on the adverse effects of proton pump inhibitors (PPIs), I strongly support the attached petition for Black Box Warnings and other labeling changes to the labels of all PPIs currently on the market and have joined Public Citizen as a co-petitioner.

My research began in 1974 on the regulation of gastric acid secretion, and particularly the central role of gastrin in this process. Through *in vitro* studies in isolated organs, in addition to *in vivo* animal and, most importantly human studies, our group was the first to show that gastrin, a critical hormone in regulating digestion, functionally stimulates acid secretion primarily through effects on histamine release. A key finding was that, once the PPIs were discontinued, ECL cell hyperplasia persisted for weeks and even a few months causing levels of acid secretion higher than those seen before starting PPI therapy.

From these initial animal data on the effect of PPIs on gastrin with secondary ECL cell hyperplasia, it was difficult to accept that these drugs should not induce a rebound acid hypersecretion (RAHS) in humans, and in a 1996 study on patients with reflux esophagitis, we were the first to show such an effect. We reasoned that this RAHS effect was the cause of the "dependence" on PPIs that many clinicians in the field have described. As outlined in the petition, our findings have been confirmed by a wave of subsequent studies showing, in randomized-controlled trials, that patients with gastroesophageal reflux disease (GERD) can become "dependent" on PPIs through the RAHS effect after as little as 2 weeks of therapy. In 2009 in another randomized trial, even previously healthy subjects – with no history of GERD – showed the RAHS effect after two weeks of PPI therapy, thus confirming that the effect is not merely a recurrence of symptoms after stopping therapy.

This area of research has become increasingly important since the proliferation of PPI use over the past 10-15 years to become one of the most widely used classes of medications in the world. However, throughout my career I have been struck by the difficulties in getting manuscripts published describing this and other adverse effects of PPIs. Furthermore, it has been disappointing to experience that clinicians and scientists dismiss the alteration by PPIs of central biological functions and believe that some of these basic functions can be removed without consequences.

For instance, one of the most important functions of the acidic gastric juice is to kill swallowed micro-organisms. Thus, by suppressing gastric acid secretion and removing this critical protective mechanism against infection, PPIs have been shown to increase the risk of several infections, such as pneumonia and *C. difficile* diarrhea. This represents just one of many life-threatening side effects that have been associated with long-term PPI use. In addition, several animal studies have shown a possible link between PPI use and gastric cancer, particularly in patients with a common stomach infection, *H. pylori*, the same bacteria implicated in peptic ulcer disease.

Given that most people on PPIs long-term do not even have a documented need for the medication, and that for those that are on these drugs for legitimate reasons, several safer alternatives exist, the risks greatly outweigh any benefit in most patients on PPIs. I therefore urge the FDA to act promptly on the recommendations outlined in Public Citizen's petition to require urgent labeling changes to all PPIs, including Black Box Warnings describing these serious adverse effects.

Sincerely,

Helge L. Waldum, M.D., PhD,
Professor of Medicine and Head of Department of Digestive and Liver Diseases
Norwegian National University of Science and Technology
Trondheim University Hospital
N-7006
Trondheim, Norway

Petition on PPI Adverse Effects Prompts Discussion

Public Citizen asks FDA for boxed warnings on all PPIs, but the evidence is inadequate, others say.

BY ELIZABETH MECHCATIE
Elsevier Global Medical News

In August, the consumer advocacy group Public Citizen filed a citizen's petition with the FDA asking that the agency require boxed warnings on the labels of all prescription proton pump inhibitors (PPIs) regarding the risk of fractures and other adverse events.

The petition, a 39-page document that includes 183 footnotes, cites the increasing popularity of PPIs during the past 20 years, their "massive inappropriate use," and safety problems that Public Citizen alleges are associated with long-term use of PPIs. The petition states that up to two-thirds of people taking a PPI "do not have a verified indication for the drug," citing a 2009 study, and also refers to the potential for developing "dependence" on PPIs resulting in rebound hypersecretion of stomach acid.

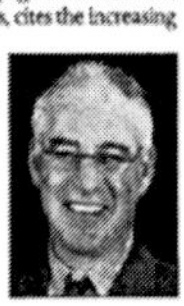

A boxed warning is not warranted for PPIs, but physicians should prescribe the lowest effective maintenance dose.

DR. METZ

Public Citizen also stated that in addition to the increased risk for hip, spine, and wrist fractures, the list of risks should include rebound acid hypersecretion (not mentioned in current labels); *Clostridium difficile* and other serious infections; and "magnesium deficiency" – with "equivalent, prominent warnings" about these risks on labels for over-the-counter PPIs.

Currently, none of the approved PPIs has a boxed warning, and the risks of fractures and hypomagnesemia (not magnesium deficiency) are listed in the highlights section of the labels, while information on *C. difficile* infections is only included in the labels of three PPIs. The petition also asks the FDA to require other labeling changes about drug-drug interactions, namely, that PPIs may reduce the effectiveness of clopidogrel; the potential for vitamin B-12 deficiency with long-term PPI use; and the potential for drug-induced interstitial nephritis that has been described in at least 60 case reports, according to the petition.

The interaction with clopidogrel is included in the omeprazole label, since that is one of the PPIs that has been shown to be more likely to interact with clopidogrel than others, but the petition argues that the highlights section of all PPIs should include the statement that "the potential for a classwide interaction cannot be ruled out at this time."

The petition also states that it is "biologically plausible" that long-term therapy with proton pump inhibitors could lead to development of gastric carcinoid tumors, a specific type of stomach cancer. And the petition calls for the addition of specific recommendations on treatment duration to the indication sections of the labels for all PPIs approved for treating gastroesophageal reflux disease (GERD).

Public Citizen's petition also urges the FDA to require that patients be given a medication guide with all prescriptions for PPIs, including refills, with information on the adverse effect warnings and alternatives to PPIs, and for all manufacturers to send a health care practitioner letter "alerting physicians to these adverse effects and to include information on appropriate prescribing of PPIs in inpatient and outpatient settings."

In a statement issued on August 23 announcing that the petition had been filed with the FDA, Dr. Sidney Wolfe, director of Public Citizen's Health Research Group, called on the agency to "act immediately to ensure that patients and physicians are adequately warned of these effects, and reminded of the many safer alternatives for common conditions such as acid reflux."

"It is critical that these potentially dangerous adverse effects be made known to the public since they pose a serious threat to the general well-being of PPI users," the statement says. "The added risk information, and provider and patient awareness of appropriate PPI use, should help to limit the massive amount of needless overprescribing."

In an interview, Dr. David C. Metz, AGAF, professor of medicine and associate chief for clinical affairs in the division of gastroenterology, University of Pennsylvania, Philadelphia, said he does not believe a boxed warning is warranted for proton pump inhibitors. As with all prescription medications, the use of PPIs for acid suppression has certain clinical indications and potential risks, and there are reasons why acid suppression should be considered, he said.

"Our job is to prescribe appropriate medications for use by our patients with the understanding of the risk-benefit assessment," he said in an interview. "Adding a boxed warning about the potential risks of PPIs would be like adding a boxed warning to antibiotics stating that occasionally, people have a fatal allergic reaction."

While he disagrees with the need for a boxed warning, he does believe that an important message for clinicians is to use the lowest effective dose of a PPI, when a PPI is indicated long-term. "The mantra should be the lowest effective maintenance dose," which depends on the indication, he said, noting that a twice daily dose or even a once daily dose may not be necessary and that a dose every other day may be adequate for some patients. This is an important message for clinicians, but does not require a boxed warning, he said.

For example, a patient with Barrett's esophagus, whether symptomatic or asymptomatic, should be on a PPI at least once a day, while a patient with reflux who does not have Barrett's should be on the lowest effective dose, which might be less than once a day. "There's a general misperception among gastroenterologists that two is better than one without much data to prove it," he remarked.

Dr. Metz also agrees that PPIs are overused in several areas, and that twice-a-day dosing is used more often than necessary, but said that for every patient Public Citizen says is overtreated with a PPI, there are "many, many" patients who should be receiving a PPI but are not, most importantly, patients on NSAIDs, who should be treated with a PPI.

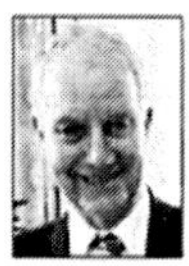

'It has been sad to notice that the respect for biological function [gastric acid secretion] has been so low.'

DR. WALDUM

NSAIDs – including even low-dose aspirin – can cause fatal upper GI bleeding, especially in elderly patients, and the risk factors are well understood. The risk can be largely mitigated (by 50% or so) by co-prescribing at-risk individuals with a PPI, Dr. Metz said. "This is very beneficial and I am personally concerned that by painting all PPI users with the same brush we run the potential risk of exposing NSAID patients to increased risks by withholding therapy when indicated," he added.

Citing numerous animal studies, Public Citizen's petition states that it is "biologically plausible" that long-term PPI treatment could result in the development of gastric carcinoid tumors, since long-term acid suppression is a major cause of hypergastrinemia, and a hypergastrinemic state induces enterochromaffin-like (ECL) cell changes. It also says that ECL cell changes "are thought to progress through hyperplastic and dysplastic states before finally becoming carcinoids." The petition also cites studies that "strengthen the likelihood that gastrin-induced ECL cell hyperplasia resulting from PPI therapy" is the cause of rebound acid hypersecretion, and that lowering gastric acidity with PPI treatment could improve the survival of the organism *C. difficile*.

While noting that the concept of rebound acid hypersecretion is currently a controversial topic with mixed results in research studies, Dr. Metz said, "personally, I think rebound is a real phenomenon and that's why I favor the lowest effective maintenance dose." Rebound is dependent on duration and dose of PPI treatment, so the longer a patient is on a PPI and the higher the dose, the more likely rebound will occur if treatment is stopped, Dr. Metz added.

The reason why long-term acid suppression can potentially predispose patients to rebound hypersecretion when the PPI is withdrawn is that serum gastrin increases during long-term acid suppression, he said. While he would not use the term "dependence" to describe this – the petition refers to hypergastrinemia and symptomatic rebound acid hypersecretion as "a form of dependence" on PPIs – he does believe that an excessive dose for a long period of time predisposes patients to this phenomenon and that using the lowest effective maintenance dose will have less of an impact on the gastrin drive and will reduce the risk of rebound.

Dr. Metz is the author of a recently published study that did not find evidence of rebound in patients on a PPI. However, in two other recent studies in healthy volunteers, a possible rebound effect was documented once subjects stopped receiving the PPI (Reimer et al., Gastroenterology 2009;137:80-7; and Niklasson et al., Am. J. Gastroenterol. 2010;105:1531-7).

Common clinical scenarios in which PPIs are overused, Dr. Metz said, include patients who are put on a PPI twice a day for a little bit of discomfort that is not true reflux, and people who are prescribed a PPI in the hospital for "stress ulcer prophylaxis" but are not taken off the PPI when they move from a critical care unit to a regular unit or at discharge. Another scenario he described is when a 6-week trial of a PPI is not stopped after 6 weeks, and people who may not have a true indication for a PPI continue treatment long term.

As for the reports of an increased risk of fractures associated with PPI use, Dr. Metz said that they are based on epidemiological studies with possible confounding factors and small odds ratios, and whether PPIs retard calcium absorption is not proven. He has had patients come in with complaints of heartburn after having stopped taking the PPI because they were worried about the fracture risk. "But if patients need the drug, they should take the drug," Dr. Metz said. "These are medical decisions that should be made between the patient and the doctor. This requires an informed physician who knows the risks and benefits," he added.

In an interview, a co-petitioner with Public Citizen, Dr. Helge Waldum, head of the department of digestive and liver

Continued on following page

CORRESPONDENCE

The GI & HEPATOLOGY NEWS Board of Editors welcomes comments and opinions on GI & HEPATOLOGY NEWS and AGA activities from readers for possible publication in a new correspondence section. Letters should include your name and address, affiliation, and any conflicts of interest regarding the topics discussed. Letters may be edited for space and clarity. Submit comments to **ginews@gastro.org**.

Continued from previous page

diseases at Trondheim University in Norway and the author of the first study to report the rebound effect, emphasized the problem of PPI overuse. A PPI may not be indicated for most people currently on long-term PPI treatment, and there are safer alternatives for patients who are on a PPI for a legitimate reason, such as a histamine-2 blocker and antacids, for the mildest cases, he said.

Dr. Waldum said that physicians and patients should be more aware of the long-term problems associated with ongoing PPI treatment, which he said include an increased risk of carcinoid tumors induced by hypergastrinemia – as described in Public Citizen's petition. This risk is not appreciated by clinicians, who have a lack of biological knowledge, he said, noting that suppressing acid should not be considered similar to reducing blood pressure in a hypertensive patient.

For almost 40 years, he has conducted research on gastrin, including studies on the main biological function of gastric juice, namely the killing of swallowed microorganisms. "We have shown that PPI dosing of rodents increases the risk of prion infection when scrapie-infected sheep brain is introduced into the stomach by gavage," Dr. Waldum said.

"Throughout my career, it has been sad to notice that the respect for biological function (in the case of gastric acid secretion) has been so low that doctors have thought that it could be taken away without problems," which he said is based on the experience of patients with atrophic gastritis (pernicious anemia). But this is a disease that starts in middle age or late in life, "and is accompanied with a risk of gastric carcinomas originating from the target cell (the ECL cell) of gastrin, and an increased risk of gastrointestinal infections," he added, citing a study published in 2002 (APMIS 2002;110:132-39; http://onlinelibrary.wiley.com/doi/10.1034/j.1600-0463.2002.100302.x/abstract).

More recently, Dr. Waldum and his associates reported what he said was the first case of gastric carcinoma developing from the ECL cell in a patient with hypergastrinemia secondary to long-term PPI treatment (more than 15 years), he said (in press, Scand. J. Gastroenterol.). "Taking into consideration that our hospital is serving a population of about 600,000, I suspect that many must have seen similar cases without getting the correct diagnosis from the pathologist and thus missing the connection with the drug treatment," he said.

A spokesperson for the FDA said the agency cannot comment on the specifics of a petition letter or how the agency might respond. Regulations require that the agency provide a response to a citizen's petition within 180 days after it is received, and the response options are to approve the petition, deny it, or "provide a tentative response, indicating why the agency has been unable to reach a decision." The FDA spokesperson said that in many cases, a tentative response is issued, which satisfies the 180-day deadline, and there is no other deadline for the FDA to act, even with a tentative response.

Dr. Metz has had a consultancy agreement with Takeda in the last year, in the writing of the study cited above, and is in the process of renewing a consultancy agreement with the company. He has been a consultant, has done studies for, and/or received grant support from all PPI manufacturers in the past, but not for at least a year, with the exception of Takeda. Dr. Waldum said that he has no disclosures.

Public Citizen's petition to the FDA is available at www.citizen.org/documents/1964.pdf ■

COMMENTARY

Experts Share Their Perspectives on PPI Risks, Benefits

Dr. David A. Peura, AGAF, Professor Emeritus, University of Virginia, Charlottesville

PPIs have proven to be safe, effective, and beneficial for millions of GERD sufferers over the past 2 decades. The absolute risk and incidence of clinically important adverse events associated with their use remains very low – and PPI safety issues are already well communicated in the general product labels. Public Citizen's petition for a black box warning for PPIs is misguided, since such a warning should be reserved for serious drug-associated adverse events that are supported by high-quality clinical data. Manifestly, this is not the case for PPIs. The proposed black box warning would unnecessarily scare consumers, patients, and prescribers. It might also promote the use of less effective GERD medications, such as H_2-receptor antagonists (H_2RAs), and encourage more risky and needless antireflux surgery.

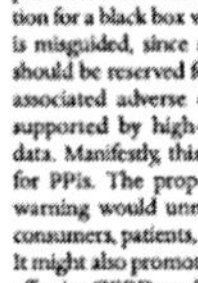

DR. DAVID A. PEURA, AGAF

Public Citizen's concerns about PPI overuse – and high-dose and prolonged use – could be better and more positively addressed by advocating for research to better understand and define the impact of their concerns. Information regarding the true extent and reasons for overuse and the need for prolonged PPI use is required before these issues can be appropriately addressed. Investigation evaluating on-demand or short-course PPI treatment (common practices among our patients) is also important since it could lead to new labeled indications for the drug class and promote more responsible use. Once this information is available, advocating for consumer, patient, and prescriber education would be the next logical and positive step to promote evidenced-based best practices that are supported by good science. Isn't this preferable to the current attempt to unnecessarily scare PPI users and prescribers, an approach that can only have negative downstream consequences?

DR. PEURA *serves as a consultant to, and is on the speaker's bureau of, PPI manufacturers.*

Dr. Richard H. Hunt, AGAF, Professor of Medicine, McMaster University, Hamilton, Ontario

The request to the FDA by Public Citizen to change the labels on PPIs to include a black box warning is of concern. If Public Citizen believes that a change is required, they should request that the FDA review the evidence regarding the safety of this drug class.

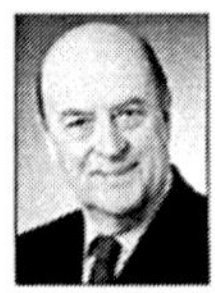

DR. RICHARD H. HUNT, AGAF

The FDA is equipped and empowered to critically review the totality of the evidence that addresses both the clinical benefits and the adverse effects. The evidence – such as is provided by Public Citizen and Professor Waldum – is incomplete, largely anecdotal, and at best weak. Their concern for all drugs to be safe must be applauded, but the PPIs have been available for more than 20 years and have brought enormous benefit to millions of patients worldwide with improved quality of life and the treatment or prevention of life-threatening events, all with a remarkable overall safety record.

Moreover, the benefits of PPIs continue to accrue in patients such as those at risk of NSAID-associated upper GI ulcers and bleeding. Indeed, the major concern should be that there are many patients who should be taking these drugs but are not doing so because of exaggerated concerns over safety, or lack of knowledge. The efforts of Public Citizen and Prof. Waldum are misdirected since they are concerned with overuse. Rather than requesting that the drugs be given a black box warning, they should be seeking better public education and physician prescribing.

Prof. Waldum's concerns over the risk of acid suppression perhaps leading to gastric cancer originated with the H_2-receptor antagonists (H_2RAs), which were launched in the late 1970s. There have been many studies and large, evidence-based focus group meetings that have examined this issue in depth and found no evidence to support the hypothetical concerns. Despite Prof. Waldum's longstanding concerns about PPIs, there have been no changes to the product information labels in his native Norway.

The more recent concern over rebound acid hypersecretion with the PPIs is less supported on a biological basis than it is for the H_2RAs, where the clinical relevance is minimal. The evidence for rebound with PPIs is controversial, with many of the claims coming from indirect evidence and questionable methodology. A systematic review on this topic found the studies controversial, with more evidence against rebound than for it. Moreover, the relationship between gastric secretory capacity and symptoms has always been questionable. In any event, the statistically small differences do not imply clinical significance, which has never been convincingly shown.

With respect to the several other concerns expressed by Public Citizen, the evidence quoted comes from a series of large observational studies. It has become common practice to trawl through large data sets in the hope of finding something. The questions may lack biological plausibility and studies suffer from poor methodology – biased data and confounding provide weak evidence.

Most importantly, observational studies do not prove causality. Not surprisingly, the finding of an increase in risk associated with PPIs from observational studies is commonly seen in patients who already suffer significant co-morbidity. Although most studies attempt to correct for this, this is very difficult, and PPI use appears to be a marker for poor health. This needs careful consideration in the interpretation of concerns about, for example, *C. difficile* infection and hip fracture. As in most indications, the benefits clearly outweigh the risks associated with these drugs.

DR. HUNT *provides clinical care for and studies patients with acid-related diseases and has been an investigator, consultant, and speaker for many of the companies developing antisecretory drugs to manage these diseases.*

Dr. James W. Freston, AGAF, Professor Emeritus, University of Connecticut, Farmington

The proposed boxed warning for PPIs is misguided. Such warnings have been and remain reserved for serious safety issues that are based on the best available evidence. The impact of the boxed warning is devalued if, as proposed by Public Citizen, these warnings are based on conflicting epidemiological associations with low odds ratios, which are by their nature confounded by alternative explanations. The fundamental fact that associations do not establish causality seems to be overlooked by Public Citizen. "Biological plausibility" is not evidence either. If

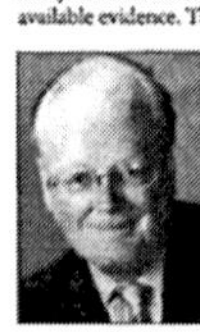

DR. JAMES W. FRESTON, AGAF

Continued on following page

18 UPPER GI TRACT

DECEMBER 2011 • GI & HEPATOLOGY NEWS

Continued from previous page

it were, we may not have had H_2-receptor antagonists (H_2RAs) today, since Dr. Wolfe of Public Citizen had advocated against FDA approval of cimetidine because of concerns of cancer risk based on the finding of testicular adenomas in rats dosed with the drug. The risk that it might do so in humans seemed biologically plausible to him.

Likewise, the relationship between elevated serum gastrin levels and gastric carcinoids (not mid-gut carcinoids or carcinomas) was established in rats over 2 decades ago. Long-term studies in man have not shown the progression of ECL cell hyperplasia to neoplasia, demonstrating yet again that rats are unlike man despite "biological plausibility." Millions of patients have been treated with PPIs over the past 15 years. We have seen no evidence of gastric carcinoids or carcinomas linked to PPIs. The excuse that "it's too soon to be sure" could be said of any drug approved in the last 3 decades.

Risk-benefit assessment is fundamental to sound prescribing. The proposed boxed warning is also ill-advised because it ignores the benefit part of risk-benefit, especially for GERD, versus so-called "safer alternatives" such as H_2RAs and antacids. The superior efficacy of PPIs is based on the highest level of evidence – namely, numerous large, randomized, double-blinded clinical trials. In the early years of the PPIs, most of my GERD patients turned to them because they suffered despite taking antacids, H_2RAs, metoclopramide, or cisapride (since withdrawn due to fatal cardiac arrhythmias), often in combination. It would be unfortunate if an initiative like Public Citizen's caused prescribers to switch back to metoclopramide, whose serious neurotoxicity dwarfs PPI safety issues in both frequency and severity.

The situation seems analogous to the widespread use of antibiotics for nonindicated conditions, such as viral infections. Some antibiotics occasionally cause severe allergic reactions and even fatal acute liver failure. Should all antibiotics also have boxed warnings? Again, this devalues the impact and utility of such warnings.

DR. FRESTON has been a consultant to companies that produce H_2RAs and PPIs until 2 years ago.

Dr. John M. Inadomi, AGAF, Professor of Medicine, University of Washington, Seattle

Public Citizen's petition to the FDA for a black box warning for PPIs is seriously misguided. This is not the first time that the PPIs have been under fire, as omeprazole originally carried a black box warning for carcinoid tumors, but this was revoked after no case of tumor was ever ascribed to PPI use. The petitioners have not learned from this past mistake, since the purported adverse events have only very weak evidence of support. This is in contrast to the very-high-quality evidence supporting the benefits of PPI use in peptic ulcer and GERD. The purported risk of increased cardiovascular events with clopidogrel is based on weak, retrospective evidence, while the highest-quality evidence, namely a randomized controlled clinical trial, demonstrates that there was no increase in cardiovascular events or mortality.

For the majority of the other proposed adverse events, primary studies as well as meta-analyses have revealed a great deal of statistical heterogeneity, which means that the data are inconsistent and are likely to be highly biased. From a clinical and therapeutic perspective, the interpretation is that the "hypotheses" developed from these low-quality studies have yet to be tested in prospective clinical trials. Certainly this effort to reclassify the risk of PPIs is not only premature but also has a high likelihood of proving to be untrue.

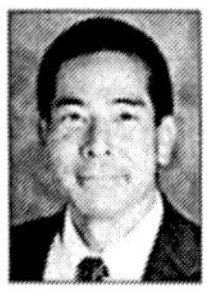

DR. JOHN M. INADOMI, AGAF

Thus, a black box warning for PPIs would be a grave mistake. Not only may it result in no change in adverse events, but it could actually cause harm to patients who would otherwise benefit from the proven effects of PPIs.

DR. INADOMI is a consultant to AstraZeneca and Takeda.

Dr. Grigoris I. Leontiadis, Assistant Professor, McMaster University, Hamilton, Ontario

Public Citizen's petition for FDA black box warnings for PPIs because of a series of alleged risks may paradoxically harm the very patients it aims to protect, and undermines the trustworthiness of future FDA black box warnings. The evidence for these risks is very weak at best; such warnings would unjustifiably reduce PPI prescribing and adherence among patients for whom there is high-quality evidence that PPIs prevent life-threatening complications (for NSAID users who have a high risk for upper GI complications) or restore quality of life (for patients such as those with GERD).

The issue of rebound acid hypersecretion is still under investigation. The current evidence is controversial, and the clinical importance and duration of the effects are questionable. Nevertheless, this research question could be easily and fairly quickly resolved by conducting one or two appropriately designed randomized, controlled trials. Therefore, it would be prudent to wait before rushing to conclusions. In any case, this risk would not justify a black box warning, which by definition is reserved for fatal, life-threatening, or permanently disabling adverse reactions.

Regarding the other alleged risks (e.g., fractures, infections, hypomagnesemia) and the suggested risk of adverse cardiovascular events due to an interaction with clopidogrel, the evidence is very fragile. Observational studies have shown weak associations, which do not prove causation. For most of these associations, several meta-analyses have invariably demonstrated unexplained statistical heterogeneity and high risk of bias among the included studies, mainly due to residual confounding. The overall strength of evidence assessed with the GRADE approach is "very low," which means that "any estimate of effect is very uncertain."

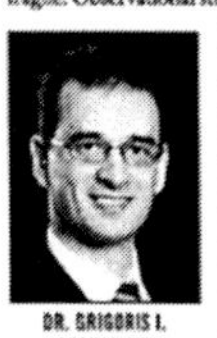

DR. GRIGORIS I. LEONTIADIS

In these observational studies, the poorer the health status of a patient, the more likely he or she was to be prescribed a PPI. All the above alleged adverse outcomes are known to occur more often among patients with poor health status and comorbidities. Most of the studies have attempted to adjust for comorbidity as a confounding factor, but the identification and quantification of comorbidity was inevitably crude, given the design of the studies.

Thus it seems that PPI use is a reliable marker for poor overall health status. It is very likely that if an observational study were to assess the association between PPI use and herpes zoster (or any other disease that is expected to occur more often in people with poor health status), it would also show a statistically significant "association." Evidence-based medicine and, most importantly, common sense will hopefully prevail.

DR. LEONTIADIS has been a consultant to a PPI manufacturer in the past, but not for at least 2 years.

Dr. M. Michael Wolfe, AGAF, Chair, Case Western Reserve University Department of Medicine at MetroHealth Medical Center, Cleveland

PPIs are among the most widely prescribed medications in the world and have been used in the United States for the past 22 years by tens of millions of individuals. Prior to their development, the only medical therapy available for treating GERD and other acid-related disorders was the histamine H_2-receptor antagonists (H_2RAs). Despite their marked benefit in the treatment of peptic ulcer and mild episodic heartburn, H_2RAs have proven largely ineffective for treating esophagitis and other more severe forms of GERD. The availability of PPIs has improved the quality of life for countless individuals and revolutionized the treatment of GERD.

It must be emphasized that GERD is not a trivial medical disorder. Not only is quality of life adversely affected, but GERD may also be associated with serious complications. For example, since the introduction of PPIs, studies have shown that the incidence of peptic esophageal strictures has diminished dramatically. Moreover, these agents constitute the only effective form of medical therapy for treating Barrett's esophagus, a premalignant condition of the esophagus associated with long-standing reflux disease. Meanwhile, the most rapidly increasing malignancy in the United States and other Western nations is esophageal adenocarcinoma in the setting of Barrett's esophagus.

Every drug used to treat human disease possesses the capacity to produce potential adverse effects, and it is imperative that risk/benefit analyses be performed before instituting any form of therapy. In this regard, the therapeutic index of PPIs is among the widest of all classes of medication. Many of the purported adverse properties attributed to PPIs have not been confirmed, and some are questionable.

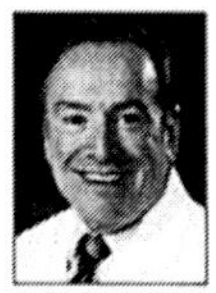

DR. M. MICHAEL WOLFE, AGAF

For example, it is difficult to mechanistically attribute an increase in *Clostridium difficile* infection to the suppression of acid secretion by PPIs when the organism is transmitted by acid-resistant spores. Rather, this purported adverse property may be artifactual and potentially attributable to the use of PPIs in individuals with more serious systemic diseases. Moreover, the interaction with clopidogrel has not been detected in all studies.

Nevertheless, patients and physicians must be aware of potential adverse properties of any medication. The inclusion of "black box" warnings is unwarranted and may actually be deleterious to many individuals, who may unnecessarily discontinue their medication and thereby exacerbate their acid-related condition and potentially expose themselves to the development of serious complications.

All medication should be used judiciously and at the lowest effective dose, particularly if used for prolonged periods of time. PPIs are no different in this regard. Physician and patient education programs have proven invaluable in ensuring the appropriate use of PPIs and should continue, particularly in light of concerns raised by citizen advocacy groups. These educational efforts, rather than instilling fear, represent the optimal means for achieving such desired goals.

DR. WOLFE is not a consultant, and is not on the speakers' bureau, of any PPI manufacturers. He was Chair of the FDA Advisory Board for GI Drugs, invented Pepcid Complete, and wrote a book for the public on reflux disease, "Heartburn: Extinguishing The Fire Inside."

What can be done?

My intention with this short book is to show that you may encounter commercial interests at any level of medical science. Moreover, all parts of medical research may have clinical consequences, and thus have a potential economic impact. Everybody has an interest in detecting short-term side effects and complications, but it becomes particularly problematic when dealing with long-term risks. Malignant tumors occur mainly in the elderly, because neoplasia takes time to develop. Until recently, evaluating the risk of a new drug inducing neoplasia was based upon toxicity studies in small animals with a short life span.

This principle was not followed when the first PPI, omeprazole, was accepted for clinical use despite causing malignant tumors in its target organ, the oxyntic mucosa of the stomach. This had not happened before. The argument for breaking the old taboo and allowing the clinical use of a compound causing neoplasia in animals, was that the tumors that had occurred in the rats were particular to that species. Moreover, omeprazole was initially only accepted for use in severe peptic ulcer disease, including gastrinomas.

However, over time, the use of PPIs has spread to all degrees of dyspeptic complaints since they often have a long-term good symptomatic effect and apparently few side effects. Therefore, PPIs are among the most used drugs, and their producers have earned a lot of money. However, it is not true that ECL cell derived tumors, which are secondary to long-term hypergastrinemia, are only found in rats. It has often been overlooked that PPIs induce tumors, not directly via their compounds, but because of their biological effect: the inhibition of acid secretion. Thus, the lack of tumors in mice who had been dosed with PPIs (Ekman et al. 1985) only reflects that the mice are very resistant to the acid inhibitory effect of PPIs, and it does not prove that hypergastrinemia does not induce ECL tumors in that species. In fact, histamine-2 blockers are efficient inhibitors of acid secretion in mice, and they also induce ECL cell derived tumors from hypergastrinemia in them (Poynter et al. 1986).

Similarly, Astra dosed dogs with PPIs to a high level without seeing any signs of tumors (Safholm et al. 1994), leading them to claim that ECL cell tumors due to long-term use of inhibitors of acid secretion only occur in rodents. Again, however, the dose of the PPI used, although high, did not inhibit acid secretion, and so there was no hypergastrinemia. This canine study does not say anything about the risk of PPI use in humans, where the doses given have a marked and sustained hypoacidity and, therefore, appreciable hypergastrinemia. However, it must be admitted that the species' eating habits probably will have an influence on the degree of 24h gastrinemia. Thus, species like rodents, who have a stomach full of food all the time, will probably have higher gastrin values than dogs, who only eat once a day. Humans are, in this respect, between rodents and dogs. In all the species studied, long-term hypergastrinemia induced ECL cell derived tumors. It has been known for many years that PPI treatment induces ECL cell hyperplasia in humans(Lamberts et al. 1988) , which is the initial ECL change observed in rodents prior to manifesting neoplasia. In fact, any condition with long-term hypergastrinemia in any species that has been studied, gives rise to ECL cell derived tumors of variable degrees of malignancy.

Moreover, the first ECL cell carcinoids secondary to PPIs have now been described (Jianu et al. 2012; Cavalcoli et al. 2015). Given the huge and long-term use of PPIs, there is every reason to fear that we will see many more tumors in the future.

How did the widespread use of PPIs occur?

The main reason was that Astra managed to make the medical community accept that the occurrence of ECL cell tumors secondary to PPI dosing in rats was not relevant for humans.

Instead, relying on so-called evidence-based medicine, PPIs were shown to be efficient and safe in short-term studies. By convincing medical experts and medical authorities that treatment should be based on evidence-based medicine, doctors started to use PPIs on a large scale to treat rather commonplace symptoms.

In terms of the risk of neoplasia, these studies are of little value. However, in humans the first stage, like in rodent ECL cell neoplasia development, is ECL cell hyperplasia, which was described shortly after entering PPIs into clinical use. It should be recalled that humans and rats are more than 90% genetically similar. Therefore, we should stick to the custom of avoiding using drugs that cause malignant diseases in laboratory animals to treat benign diseases. If we had continued to use PPIs only in patients suffering from severe acid-related disease, which was the original purpose of omeprazole, the use of PPIs would have been justified. Moreover, since ECL cell carcinogenesis takes time, such drugs can be used more liberally in elderly people.

How do we prevent widespread use of drugs that may cause serious diseases in the future?

The most important thing is not to rely on evidence-based medicine alone, since long-term side effects/complications cannot be detected by these types of studies.

Only long-term animal studies can give an indication of this type of toxicity. Moreover, when the toxicity is not a direct effect of the compound, but a consequence of its biological effects, studies that do not engage with this cannot say anything about the level of risk.

I will also add that the authorities should look at the personal benefits of those giving positive statements versus the ones coming up with negative statements about a compound.

Finally, I have frequently mentioned AstraZeneca in relation to PPIs because this is my area of clinical and scientific experience. However, I do not believe that AstraZeneca is worse than other companies, although it was the first one to make medical experts accept a compound (omeprazole) that induces malignant tumors in its target organ in a small animal (rat) after long-term dosing for use on humans. This means that the development of neoplasia in small animals does not preclude clinical use.

Postscript

The previous chapters were written more than three years ago. I did not attempt to publish them at that time, out of fear of being sued. During the last few years, there has been a marked change in the attitudes towards PPI side effects. Thus, there have been reports incriminating the use of PPIs in the development of different diseases, such as cardiac disease (Shih et al. 2014), cerebrovascular disease (Wang et al. 2017), dementia (Gomm et al. 2016), and kidney diseases (Klatte et al. 2017). For most of these diseases, there was an increased risk in PPI users compared to non-users, although the mechanisms behind these side effects have not been stated. For dementia, however, we proposed that it could be related to prion infections (H. L. Waldum and Martinsen 2016), since the inhibition of gastric acid secretion makes mice more susceptible to prion infections (Martinsen et al. 2002; Martinsen et al. 2011). Nevertheless, there has been no plausible mechanism found behind the other putative side effects, and it is impossible to avoid suspecting that they reflect confounding factors, although the authors have tried to exclude them. However, on October, 31, 2017, two papers were published describing an increased incidence of gastric cancer in patients taking PPIs (Cheung et al. 2018; Brusselaers et al. 2017). In particular, the study from Hong Kong, which described an increased incidence of gastric cancer in the follow-up after the eradication of Helicobacter pylori in patients using PPIs compared to non-users (Cheung et al. 2018), seems convincing and has also been confirmed (Peng et al. 2019). The other was a Swedish epidemiological study, which was based upon a drug register and a cancer register (both of a high quality); this showed an increased incidence of gastric cancer in patients taking PPIs after the removal of known confounding factors (Brusselaers et al. 2017). There is reason to assume that the gastric carcinogenic factor caused by PPI use is hypergastrinemia. A study from Finland described how people with elevated gastrin levels had an increased risk of developing gastric cancer over time (Murphy et al. 2017). It seems, therefore, that PPI treatment leads to an increased risk of gastric cancer. This has not been detected before, because carcinogenesis takes decades to develop. Parallel to the introduction of PPIs to the market the decline in the Helicobacter pylori (the most important gastric carcinogen) infection rate has continued. Interestingly, the gastric carcinogenic effect of Helicobacter pylori infection may be due to hypergastrinemia secondary to reduced acid secretion from atrophic gastritis (H. L. Waldum et al. 2015). Moreover, the carcinogenic effect of PPI treatment that has been recorded in patients after Helicobacter pylori has been eradicated may reflect that both PPIs and Helicobacter pylori gastritis predispose patients to gastric cancer via gastrin (H. L. Waldum and Rehfeld 2019; H. L. Waldum, Sandvik, and Brenna 1993).

Currently, we are in an early phase of understanding the role that PPIs play in human gastric carcinogenesis. The magnitude of the problem will only become clear in the future, but there is every reason to fear that it will increase over time. The consequences of removing the gastric defense against infections via the gut, may also be significant. The recent report of the increased incidence of primary hepatic carcinoma in patients having PPI treatment (Tran et al. 2018) may be due to bacterial translocation (Llorente et al. 2017) from the removal of the gastric juices' bactericide effect. We have long stated that the gastric juice is important not only in the defense against bacterial infections, but also virus and prions(Martinsen, Bergh, and Waldum 2005). In this connection I will mention the very recent report describing that patients on PPI could have increased risk of COVID-19 infection(Almario, Chey, and Spiegel. 2020).

When taking PPIs into clinical use, two main errors were made:

1. A group of drugs causing malignant neoplasia in their target organ in animals were accepted for human use.

2. An important biological function was removed.

A very recent dispute with *Gastroenterology*

Neoplasia due to profound acid inhibition by proton pump inhibitors and a comment on a recent editorial in *Gastroenterology* claiming to represent the truth.

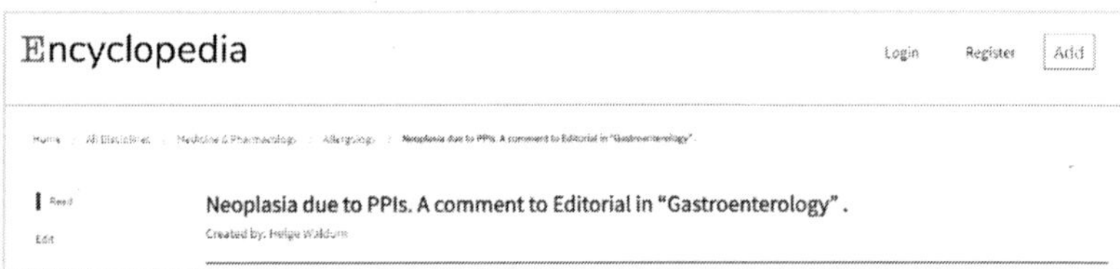

Neoplasia due to PPIs. A comment to Editorial in "Gastroenterology" .

Others

Subjects: Allergology View times: 342

Abstract

The gastric hormone gastrin is released when the gastric content acidity is too low to efficiently kill swallowed microorganisms. Gastrin stimulates the ECL cell to produce histamine which in turn stimulates the acid producing parietal cell to secrete acid. Parallel to the stimulation of the ECL cell function, gastrin also stimulates the ECL cell proliferation. Prolonged elevation of gastrin results in ECL cell hyperplasia and further to ECL cell neoplasia of varying malignancy known from about 1980. The proton pump inhibitors (PPIs) are the most efficient inhibitors of acid secretion and are very efficient in the treatment of acid related diseases or symptoms. Before their acceptance for clinical us, PPIs were known to induce neoplasia in rodents, but the medical community accepted that these tumors were not relevant for man. With time there have been accumulating evidence for PPI induced neoplasia also in man. However, very recently a large observation study financed by a pharmaceutical company, patients were followed for an average of 3 years without any evidence of neoplasia. The study was published in "Gastroenterology" and resulted in an "Editorial" claiming that the truth was approached. Unfortunately, the "Editorial " did not consider animal studies and recent studies in man reporting increased risk of gastric cancer in patients on PPI after eradication of Helicobacter pylori compared with those not taking PPI after eradication. Therefore the "Editorial" was flawed and I wrote a letter commenting on these errors. After 2 weeks I got a refusal claiming that my letter was without relevance and importance. I found that peculiar, and I also mean that a journal has an obligation to print letters showing faults with papers published and especially concerning a misleading "Editorial". I therefore publish my letter allowing others to evaluate the relevance and importance

Rejected letter to "Gastroenterology"

I read with interest and astonishment the editorial by Corley [1] based upon a multinational observational study of pantoprazole treatment compared with placebo followed for about 3 years by Moayyedi et al. [2]. They did not find evidence of any harmful effect on the kidneys or the cardiovascular system where previous epidemiological studies have suggested increased risk of disease. This was to be expected since there were no plausible mechanisms for these side effects. However, based upon the Moayyedi study Corley also seems to conclude that there is no reason to worry about neoplasia due to long-term PPI therapy. As I see it, this reflects lack of biological, physiological and pathological knowledge, because:

1: Cancer is mainly a disease of old age reflecting years of development. Three years say nothing. Children in a Spanish family with a missense mutation in one of the proton pump genes developed ECL carcinoids in their twenties and more malignant tumor in the thirties [3, 4] which is in line with the latency in animal studies done in the 1980s [5, 6]. This Spanish family is the best model for long-term PPI treatment in man and underscores that one should be particularly reluctant to put children on PPI treatment. The tumors both in the animals and the Spanish family[6 3-5] were due to hypergastrinemia secondary to hypoacidity. Moreover, Håkanson et al.[7] found that long-term PPI dosing of rats induced a positive trophic effect only in the oxyntic mucosa and particularly the ECL cell. It is therefore strange that the focus during all the years with PPIs has not been on gastric cancer [8]. Since 1990 we have published multiple studies describing ECL cell/neuroendocrine differentiation in human gastric carcinomas [8, 9]. I have wondered why pharmaceutical industry has not supported a study disapproving the role of the ECL cell in gastric carcinogenesis[10] and thus taken away an important argument for a risk of hypergastrinemia and PPI treatment. Such a study would have been much more important with respect to cancer than the Moayyedi study. In fact, to assess cancer risk we must rely on studies on animals with a much shorter life span than man. Accordingly, Moayyedi study is without value with respect to cancer.

It is also very peculiar that Helicobacter pylori (Hp) in combination with PPI treatment is not mentioned, since it is confirmed in studies from East Asia that PPI treatment after Hp eradication increases the risk of gastric cancer [11-13]. Hp gastritis is the principal cause of gastric cancer [14], and Uemura et al. showed that Hp gastritis predisposes to gastric cancer only after having induced atrophy of the oxyntic mucosa [15]. Since not only Hp oxyntic atrophic gastritis, but also autoimmune atrophic gastritis predisposes to gastric cancer [16], we have argued that Hp gastritis causes gastric cancer via hypergastrinemia [17]. Anyhow, the studies from East-Asia [11-13] cannot be dismissed.

2: Biological function of gastric juice.

The biological function of the highly acid gastric juice is to kill swallowed microorganism. In the study by Moayyedi [2] this aspect is only sparsely covered, but it seems that there was an increased risk of enteric infections[2]. We do not know the etiology of most of the chronic inflammatory diseases as well as degenerative disease of the central nervous system, but infectious agents could be the cause of many of these diseases. The gut is a possible entrance for infections by micro-organisms escaping destruction in the stomach as exemplified by poliomyelitis. Variant Creutzfeldt-Jacob disease in man due to intake of meat contaminated with pathogenic prion is another example of such a disease. In this context I will mention that we have described that mice given scrapie infected brain were more prone to develop disease when dosed with PPI [18]. It should be recalled that many infections may cause disease after decades of latency.

To conclude, for complications with a latency of decades the study by Moayyedi et al.[2]is of little value, and we must rely on biological knowledge and animal studies. The editorial by Corley lacks completely these aspects [1]. I prefer to rely more on the evolution than imperfect studies.

Trondheim August 5th, 2019

Helge L. Waldum

Professor of Medicine.

References

1.Corley DA. Safety and Complications of Long-Term Proton Pump Inhibitor Therapy: Getting Closer to the Truth. Gastroenterology 2019;157(3):604-7.2.

2. Moayyedi P, Eikelboom JW, Bosch J, et al. Safety of Proton Pump Inhibitors Based on a Large, Multi-Year, Randomized Trial of Patients Receiving Rivaroxaban or Aspirin. Gastroenterology 2019;157(3):682-91. e2.

3. Calvete O, Reyes J, Zuniga S, et al. Exome sequencing identifies ATP4A gene as responsible of an atypical familial type I gastric neuroendocrine tumour. Hum Mol Genet 2015; 24: 2914-22.

4. Fossmark R, Calvete O, Mjones P, et al. ECL-cell carcinoids and carcinoma in patients homozygous for an inactivating mutation in the gastric H (+) K (+) ATPase alpha subunit. Apmis 2016; 124:561-6.

5. Havu N. Enterochromaffin-like cell carcinoids of gastric mucosa in rats after life-long inhibition of gastric secretion. Digestion 1986;35 Suppl 1:42-55.

6. Poynter D, Selway SA, Papworth SA, et al. Changes in the gastric mucosa of the mouse associated with long lasting unsurmountable histamine H2 blockade. Gut 1986; 27: 1338-46.

7. Hakanson R, Blom H, Carlsson E, et al. Hypergastrinaemia produces trophic effects in stomach but not in pancreas and intestines. Regul Pept 1986; 13:225-33.

8. Waldum HL, Sagatun L, Mjones P. Gastrin and Gastric Cancer. Front Endocrinol (Lausanne) 2017; 8: 1.

9. Waldum HL, Fossmark R. Types of Gastric Carcinomas. Int J Mol Sci 2018; Dec 18;19(12). pii: E4109. doi: 10.3390/ijms19124109. Review.

10. Waldum HL, Sordal OF, Mjones PG. The Enterochromaffin-like [ECL] Cell-Central in Gastric Physiology and Pathology. Int J Mol Sci 2019;20. May 17;20(10). pii: E2444. doi: 10.3390/ijms20102444. Review.

11.Cheung KS, Chan EW, Wong AYS, et al. Long-term proton pump inhibitors and risk of gastric cancer development after treatment for Helicobacter pylori: a population-based study. Gut 2018; 67: 28-35.

12. Niikura R, Hayakawa Y, Hirata Y, et al. Long-term proton pump inhibitor use is a risk factor of gastric cancer after treatment for Helicobacter pylori: a retrospective cohort analysis. Gut 2018; 67: 1908-1910.

13. Lai SW, Lai HC, Lin CL, et al. Proton pump inhibitors and risk of gastric cancer in a case-control study. Gut 2019; 68: 765-767.

14. Parsonnet J, Friedman GD, Vandersteen DP, et al. Helicobacter pylori infection and the risk of gastric carcinoma. N Engl J Med 1991; 325:1127-31.

15. Uemura N, Okamoto S, Yamamoto S, et al. Helicobacter pylori infection and the development of gastric cancer. N Engl J Med 2001;345: 784-9.

16. Vannella L, Lahner E, Osborn J, et al. Systematic review: gastric cancer incidence in pernicious anaemia. Aliment Pharmacol Ther 2013; 37:375-82.

17. Waldum HL, Hauso O, Sordal OF, et al. Gastrin May Mediate the Carcinogenic Effect of Helicobacter pylori Infection of the Stomach. Dig Dis Sci 2015; 60:1522-7.

18. Martinsen TC, Benestad SL, Moldal T, et al. Inhibitors of gastric acid secretion increase the risk of prion infection in mice. Scand J Gastroenterol 2011;46: 1418-22.

I will finally add that I am not alone in being aware of the problem with commercial interests within medical science, including gastroenterology. In 2000, the current leading world-wide gastroenterologist, TC Wang, wrote an editorial with the title, "Follow the money".

Gastroenterology 2000; 118:819

Comments from the Editors

by Timothy C. Wang, Associate Editor

"Follow the Money"

In this editorial, Wang wrote that important financial conflicts of interest (both by authors and reviewers) are often not disclosed.

Moreover, physicians' monetary ties to the drug industry had led to significant bias.

Interestingly, the steady decline in the incidence in early onset (before the age of 45 years) gastric cancers showed a break in 1995, which was followed by a steady increase (Bergquist et al. 2019). At that point, PPIs had been in use for some years (H. L. Waldum 2020), which suggests a causal relationship.

Conclusion

It is to be expected that the pharmaceutical industry, like other private companies, attempts to earn as much money as possible using all available methods. In order to be balanced, academic institutions must not be dependent on the pharmaceutical industry and should instead be founded by the state. Scientific journals should not be allowed to use people who have connections to pharmaceutical industry as editors or reviewers, and they should be obliged to accept critical correspondence. Moreover, disclosing the names of the reviewers would probably increase the quality of the referee reports.

I know that every now and then most researchers become frustrated because journals do not hold the same opinions as themselves about the importance of a submitted manuscript. As an Editor-in-Chief, I know that many authors feel that they have not been treated fairly. I have tried to investigate whether I have been too sensitive. However, I cannot escape the feeling that my manuscripts have been met with a negative attitude that is peculiar, because they have later been found to be correct. Therefore, I cannot see any other possibility than non-scientific interests have been involved.

References

Almario, C.V., W.D. Chey, and B.M.R. Spiegel. 2020. "Increased risk of COVID-19 among users of proton pump inhibitors." *Am J Gastroenterol* In press.

Bakke, I., G. Qvigstad, A. K. Sandvik, and H. L. Waldum. 2001. "The CCK-2 receptor is located on the ECL cell, but not on the parietal cell." *Scand J Gastroenterol* 36 (11): 1128-33.

Bergquist, J. R., J. L. Leiting, E. B. Habermann, S. P. Cleary, M. L. Kendrick, R. L. Smoot, D. M. Nagorney, M. J. Truty, and T. E. Grotz. 2019. "Early-onset gastric cancer is a distinct disease with worrisome trends and oncogenic features." *Surgery* 166 (4): 547-555. https://doi.org/10.1016/j.surg.2019.04.036.

Berna, M. J., B. Annibale, M. Marignani, T. V. Luong, V. Corleto, A. Pace, T. Ito, D. Liewehr, D. J. Venzon, G. Delle Fave, C. Bordi, and R. T. Jensen. 2008. "A prospective study of gastric carcinoids and enterochromaffin-like cell changes in multiple endocrine neoplasia type 1 and Zollinger-Ellison syndrome: identification of risk factors." *J Clin Endocrinol Metab* 93 (5): 1582-91. https://doi.org/10.1210/jc.2007-2279.

Bjornsson, E. 2011. "It is difficult to discontinue PPI treatment in patients with GERD." *Am J Gastroenterol* 106 (2): 367-8; author reply 368. https://doi.org/10.1038/ajg.2010.402.

Bordi, C. 1988. "Carcinoid (ECL cell) tumor of the oxyntic mucosa of the stomach, a hormone dependent neoplasm?" In *Progress in Surgical Pathology*, 177-195. Field and Wood.

Brenna, E., and H. L. Waldum. 1991. "Studies of isolated parietal and enterochromaffin-like cells from the rat." *Scand J Gastroenterol* 26 (12): 1295-306.

—. 1992. "Trophic effect of gastrin on the enterochromaffin like cells of the rat stomach: establishment of a dose response relationship." *Gut* 33 (10): 1303-6.

Brusselaers, N., K. Wahlin, L. Engstrand, and J. Lagergren. 2017. "Maintenance therapy with proton pump inhibitors and risk of gastric cancer: a nationwide population-based cohort study in Sweden." *BMJ Open* 7 (10): e017739. https://doi.org/10.1136/bmjopen-2017-017739.

Cadiot, G., C. Vissuzaine, F. Potet, and M. Mignon. 1995. "Fundic argyrophil carcinoid tumor in a patient with sporadic-type Zollinger-Ellison syndrome." *Dig Dis Sci* 40 (6): 1275-8. https://doi.org/10.1007/bf02065537.

Cavalcoli, F., A. Zilli, D. Conte, C. Ciafardini, and S. Massironi. 2015. "Gastric neuroendocrine neoplasms and proton pump inhibitors: fact or coincidence?" *Scand J Gastroenterol* 50 (11): 1397-403. https://doi.org/10.3109/00365521.2015.1054426.

Cheung, K. S., E. W. Chan, A. Y. S. Wong, L. Chen, I. C. K. Wong, and W. K. Leung. 2018. "Long-term proton pump inhibitors and risk of gastric cancer development after treatment for Helicobacter pylori: a population-based study." *Gut* 67 (1): 28-35. https://doi.org/10.1136/gutjnl-2017-314605.

Dent, J., R. Jones, P. Kahrilas, and N. J. Talley. 2001. "Management of gastro-oesophageal reflux disease in general practice." *Bmj* 322 (7282): 344-7. https://doi.org/10.1136/bmj.322.7282.344.

Ekman, L., E. Hansson, N. Havu, E. Carlsson, and C. Lundberg. 1985. "Toxicological studies on omeprazole." *Scand J Gastroenterol Suppl* 108: 53-69.

Feurle, G. E. 1994. "Argyrophil cell hyperplasia and a carcinoid tumour in the stomach of a patient with sporadic Zollinger-Ellison syndrome." *Gut* 35 (2): 275-7. https://doi.org/10.1136/gut.35.2.275.

Gale, E. A. 2011. "Conflicts of interest in guideline panel members." *Bmj* 343: d5728. https://doi.org/10.1136/bmj.d5728.

Gillen, D., A. A. Wirz, J. E. Ardill, and K. E. McColl. 1999. "Rebound hypersecretion after omeprazole and its relation to on-treatment acid suppression and Helicobacter pylori status." *Gastroenterology* 116 (2): 239-47. https://doi.org/10.1016/s0016-5085(99)70118-6.

Gomm, W., K. von Holt, F. Thome, K. Broich, W. Maier, A. Fink, G. Doblhammer, and B. Haenisch. 2016. "Association of Proton Pump

Inhibitors With Risk of Dementia: A Pharmacoepidemiological Claims Data Analysis." *JAMA Neurol* 73 (4): 410-6. https://doi.org/10.1001/jamaneurol.2015.4791.

Gregory, R. A., and H. J. Tracy. 1961. "The preparation and properties of gastrin." *J Physiol* 156: 523-43. https://doi.org/10.1113/jphysiol.1961.sp006691.

Hatlebakk, J. G., F. Lerang, and B. Moum. 2010. "[Proton pump inhibitors do not cause stomach cancer]." *Tidsskr Nor Laegeforen* 130 (6): 592. https://doi.org/10.4045/tidsskr.10.0084.

Havu, N. 1986. "Enterochromaffin-like cell carcinoids of gastric mucosa in rats after life-long inhibition of gastric secretion." *Digestion* 35 Suppl 1: 42-55. https://doi.org/10.1159/000199381.

Hunfeld, N. G., W. P. Geus, and E. J. Kuipers. 2007. "Systematic review: Rebound acid hypersecretion after therapy with proton pump inhibitors." *Aliment Pharmacol Ther* 25 (1): 39-46. https://doi.org/10.1111/j.1365-2036.2006.03171.x.

Jianu, C. S., R. Fossmark, T. Viset, G. Qvigstad, O. Sordal, R. Marvik, and H. L. Waldum. 2012. "Gastric carcinoids after long-term use of a proton pump inhibitor." *Aliment Pharmacol Ther* 36 (7): 644-9. https://doi.org/10.1111/apt.12012.

Klatte, D. C. F., A. Gasparini, H. Xu, P. de Deco, M. Trevisan, A. L. V. Johansson, B. Wettermark, J. Arnlov, C. J. Janmaat, B. Lindholm, F. W. Dekker, J. Coresh, M. E. Grams, and J. J. Carrero. 2017. "Association Between Proton Pump Inhibitor Use and Risk of Progression of Chronic Kidney Disease." *Gastroenterology* 153 (3): 702-710. https://doi.org/10.1053/j.gastro.2017.05.046.

Kleveland, P. M., H. L. Waldum, and H. Larsson. 1987. "Gastric acid secretion in the totally isolated, vascularly perfused rat stomach. A selective muscarinic-1 agent does, whereas gastrin does not, augment maximal histamine-stimulated acid secretion." *Scand J Gastroenterol* 22 (6): 705-13. https://doi.org/10.3109/00365528709011147.

Lamberts, R., W. Creutzfeldt, F. Stockmann, U. Jacubaschke, S. Maas, and G. Brunner. 1988. "Long-term omeprazole treatment in man: effects on gastric endocrine cell populations." *Digestion* 39 (2): 126-35. https://doi.org/10.1159/000199615.

Larsson, H., E. Carlsson, B. Ryberg, J. Fryklund, and B. Wallmark. 1988. "Rat parietal cell function after prolonged inhibition of gastric acid secretion." *Am J Physiol* 254 (1 Pt 1): G33-9. https://doi.org/10.1152/ajpgi.1988.254.1.G33.

Liddle, R. A. 2018. "Parkinson's disease from the gut." *Brain Res* 1693 (Pt B): 201-206. https://doi.org/10.1016/j.brainres.2018.01.010.

Llorente, C., P. Jepsen, T. Inamine, L. Wang, S. Bluemel, H. J. Wang, R. Loomba, J. S. Bajaj, M. L. Schubert, M. Sikaroodi, P. M. Gillevet, J. Xu, T. Kisseleva, S. B. Ho, J. DePew, X. Du, H. T. Sorensen, H. Vilstrup, K. E. Nelson, D. A. Brenner, D. E. Fouts, and B. Schnabl. 2017. "Publisher Correction: Gastric acid suppression promotes alcoholic liver disease by inducing overgrowth of intestinal Enterococcus." *Nat Commun* 8 (1): 2137. https://doi.org/10.1038/s41467-017-01779-8.

Lorenz, W., K. Thon, H. Stoltzing, E. Neugebauer, R. Lindlar, J. Sattler, and D. Weber. 1991. "Histamine and the stomach: chemical histamine assays." *Scand J Gastroenterol Suppl* 180: 9-25. https://doi.org/10.3109/00365529109093173.

Martinsen, T. C., S. L. Benestad, T. Moldal, and H. L. Waldum. 2011. "Inhibitors of gastric acid secretion increase the risk of prion infection in mice." *Scand J Gastroenterol* 46 (12): 1418-22. https://doi.org/10.3109/00365521.2011.619277.

Martinsen, T. C., K. Bergh, and H. L. Waldum. 2005. "Gastric juice: a barrier against infectious diseases." *Basic Clin Pharmacol Toxicol* 96 (2): 94-102. https://doi.org/10.1111/j.1742-7843.2005.pto960202.x.

Martinsen, T. C., D. M. Taylor, R. Johnsen, and H. L. Waldum. 2002. "Gastric acidity protects mice against prion infection?" *Scand J Gastroenterol* 37 (5): 497-500. https://doi.org/10.1080/003655202529003017.

Murphy, G., C. C. Abnet, H. Choo-Wosoba, E. Vogtmann, S. J. Weinstein, P. R. Taylor, S. Mannisto, D. Albanes, S. M. Dawsey, J. F. Rehfeld, and N. D. Freedman. 2017. "Serum gastrin and cholecystokinin are associated with subsequent development of gastric cancer in a prospective cohort of Finnish smokers." *Int J Epidemiol* 46 (3): 914-923. https://doi.org/10.1093/ije/dyx030.

Nicholls, R. D. 1999. "Peer review under review." *Science* 286 (5446): 1853. https://doi.org/10.1126/science.286.5446.1853b.

Peng, Y. C., L. R. Huang, C. L. Lin, W. Y. Hsu, C. S. Chang, H. Z. Yeh, and C. H. Kao. 2019. "Association between proton pump inhibitors use and risk of gastric cancer in patients with GERD." *Gut* 68 (2): 374-376. https://doi.org/10.1136/gutjnl-2018-316057.

Poynter, D., S. A. Selway, S. A. Papworth, and S. R. Riches. 1986. "Changes in the gastric mucosa of the mouse associated with long lasting unsurmountable histamine H2 blockade." *Gut* 27 (11): 1338-46. https://doi.org/10.1136/gut.27.11.1338.

Prusiner, S. B. 2012. "Cell biology. A unifying role for prions in neurodegenerative diseases." *Science* 336 (6088): 1511-3.

https://doi.org/10.1126/science.1222951.
Qvigstad, G., J. S. Arnestad, E. Brenna, and H. L. Waldum. 1998. "Treatment with proton pump inhibitors induces tolerance to histamine-2 receptor antagonists in Helicobacter pylori-negative patients." *Scand J Gastroenterol* 33 (12): 1244-8. https://doi.org/10.1080/00365529850172313.
Qvigstad, G., S. Falkmer, B. Westre, and H. L. Waldum. 1999. "Clinical and histopathological tumour progression in ECL cell carcinoids ("ECLomas")." *Apmis* 107 (12): 1085-92.
Qvigstad, G., T. Qvigstad, B. Westre, A. K. Sandvik, E. Brenna, and H. L. Waldum. 2002. "Neuroendocrine differentiation in gastric adenocarcinomas associated with severe hypergastrinemia and/or pernicious anemia." *Apmis* 110 (2): 132-9. https://doi.org/10.1034/j.1600-0463.2002.100302.x.
Qvigstad, G., A. K. Sandvik, E. Brenna, S. Aase, and H. L. Waldum. 2000. "Detection of chromogranin A in human gastric adenocarcinomas using a sensitive immunohistochemical technique." *Histochem J* 32 (9): 551-6.
Reimer, C., B. Sondergaard, L. Hilsted, and P. Bytzer. 2009. "Proton-pump inhibitor therapy induces acid-related symptoms in healthy volunteers after withdrawal of therapy." *Gastroenterology* 137 (1): 80-7, 87.e1. https://doi.org/10.1053/j.gastro.2009.03.058.
Rindi, G., O. Luinetti, M. Cornaggia, C. Capella, and E. Solcia. 1993. "Three subtypes of gastric argyrophil carcinoid and the gastric neuroendocrine carcinoma: a clinicopathologic study." *Gastroenterology* 104 (4): 994-1006. https://doi.org/10.1016/0016-5085(93)90266-f.
Sachs, G., H. H. Chang, E. Rabon, R. Schackman, M. Lewin, and G. Saccomani. 1976. "A nonelectrogenic H+ pump in plasma membranes of hog stomach." *J Biol Chem* 251 (23): 7690-8.
Safholm, C., N. Havu, H. Forssell, G. Sundell, and H. Mattsson. 1994. "Effect of 7 years' daily oral administration of omeprazole to beagle dogs." *Digestion* 55 (3): 139-47. https://doi.org/10.1159/000201139.
Sandvik, A. K., H. L. Waldum, P. M. Kleveland, and B. Schulze Sognen. 1987. "Gastrin produces an immediate and dose-dependent histamine release preceding acid secretion in the totally isolated, vascularly perfused rat stomach." *Scand J Gastroenterol* 22 (7): 803-8. https://doi.org/10.3109/00365528708991918.
Sharma, B. K., R. P. Walt, R. E. Pounder, M. D. Gomes, E. C. Wood, and L. H. Logan. 1984. "Optimal dose of oral omeprazole for maximal 24 hour decrease of intragastric acidity." *Gut* 25 (9): 957-64. https://doi.org/10.1136/gut.25.9.957.

Shih, C. J., Y. T. Chen, S. M. Ou, S. Y. Li, T. J. Chen, and S. J. Wang. 2014. "Proton pump inhibitor use represents an independent risk factor for myocardial infarction." *Int J Cardiol* 177 (1): 292-7. https://doi.org/10.1016/j.ijcard.2014.09.036.

Sjoblom, S. M., P. Sipponen, S. L. Karonen, and H. J. Jarvinen. 1989. "Mucosal argyrophil endocrine cells in pernicious anaemia and upper gastrointestinal carcinoid tumours." *J Clin Pathol* 42 (4): 371-7.

Solcia, E., C. Capella, R. Fiocca, G. Rindi, and J. Rosai. 1990. "Gastric argyrophil carcinoidosis in patients with Zollinger-Ellison syndrome due to type 1 multiple endocrine neoplasia. A newly recognized association." *Am J Surg Pathol* 14 (6): 503-13.

Sørdal, Ø, G. Qvigstad, I. S. Nordrum, A. K. Sandvik, B. I. Gustafsson, and H. Waldum. 2014. "The PAS positive material in gastric cancer cells of signet ring type is not mucin." *Exp Mol Pathol* 96 (3): 274-8. https://doi.org/10.1016/j.yexmp.2014.02.008.

Talley, N. J., V. Meineche-Schmidt, P. Pare, M. Duckworth, P. Raisanen, A. Pap, H. Kordecki, and V. Schmid. 1998. "Efficacy of omeprazole in functional dyspepsia: double-blind, randomized, placebo-controlled trials (the Bond and Opera studies)." *Aliment Pharmacol Ther* 12 (11): 1055-65. https://doi.org/10.1046/j.1365-2036.1998.00410.x.

Tran, K. T., U. C. McMenamin, B. Hicks, P. Murchie, A. P. Thrift, H. G. Coleman, L. Iversen, B. T. Johnston, A. J. Lee, and C. R. Cardwell. 2018. "Proton pump inhibitor and histamine-2 receptor antagonist use and risk of liver cancer in two population-based studies." *Aliment Pharmacol Ther* 48 (1): 55-64. https://doi.org/10.1111/apt.14796.

Waldum, H. L, G Qvigstad, and E Brenna. 2003. "Omeprazole, a proton pump inhibitor." In *Predictive value of rodent forestomach and gastric neuroendocrine tumours in evaluating carcinogenic risks to humans*, 159-165. Lyon: IARC Technical Publication

Waldum, H. L. 2009. "[Proton pump inhibitors should not be sold without prescription]." *Tidsskr Nor Laegeforen* 129 (21): 2263. https://doi.org/10.4045/tidsskr.09.1066.

—. 2010. "[Proton pump inhibitors without prescription]." *Tidsskr Nor Laegeforen* 130 (10): 1014. https://doi.org/10.4045/tidsskr.10.0404.

—. 2020. "The increase in early-onset gastric carcinomas from 1995 is probably due to the introduction of proton pump inhibitors." *Surgery*. https://doi.org/10.1016/j.surg.2020.01.016.

Waldum, H. L., S. Aase, I. Kvetnoi, E. Brenna, A. K. Sandvik, U. Syversen, G. Johnsen, L. Vatten, and J. M. Polak. 1998. "Neuroendocrine differentiation in human gastric carcinoma." *Cancer* 83 (3): 435-44.

Waldum, H. L., J. S. Arnestad, E. Brenna, I. Eide, U. Syversen, and A. K. Sandvik. 1996. "Marked increase in gastric acid secretory capacity after omeprazole treatment." *Gut* 39 (5): 649-53.

Waldum, H. L., and E. Brenna. 1993. "Classification of gastric carcinomas." *Hum Pathol* 24 (1): 114-5. https://doi.org/10.1016/0046-8177(93)90074-q.

—. 2002. "Gastro-oesophageal reflux disease in general practice. Last year's guidelines are probably biased." *Bmj* 324 (7335): 485-6.

Waldum, H. L., O. A. Haugen, C. Isaksen, R. Mecsei, and A. K. Sandvik. 1991. "Enterochromaffin-like tumour cells in the diffuse but not the intestinal type of gastric carcinomas." *Eur J Gastroenterol Hepatol* 3: 245-249.

Waldum, H. L., O. Hauso, O. F. Sordal, and R. Fossmark. 2015. "Gastrin May Mediate the Carcinogenic Effect of Helicobacter pylori Infection of the Stomach." *Dig Dis Sci* 60 (6): 1522-7. https://doi.org/10.1007/s10620-014-3468-9.

Waldum, H. L., and T. C. Martinsen. 2016. "Proton Pump Inhibitors and Dementia Incidence." *JAMA Neurol* 73 (8): 1026. https://doi.org/10.1001/jamaneurol.2016.1497.

Waldum, H. L., and J. F. Rehfeld. 2019. "Gastric cancer and gastrin: on the interaction of Helicobacter pylori gastritis and acid inhibitory induced hypergastrinemia." *Scand J Gastroenterol* 54 (9): 1118-1123. https://doi.org/10.1080/00365521.2019.1663446.

Waldum, H. L., A. Sandvik, and E. Brenna. 1993. "Gastrin, the enterochromaffinlike cell, and gastric tumors." *Gastroenterology* 105 (4): 1264-6. https://doi.org/10.1016/0016-5085(93)90990-t.

Waldum, H. L., and A. K. Sandvik. 1989. "Histamine and the stomach." *Scand J Gastroenterol* 24 (2): 130-9. https://doi.org/10.3109/00365528909093027.

Wang, Y. F., Y. T. Chen, J. C. Luo, T. J. Chen, J. C. Wu, and S. J. Wang. 2017. "Proton-Pump Inhibitor Use and the Risk of First-Time Ischemic Stroke in the General Population: A Nationwide Population-Based Study." *Am J Gastroenterol* 112 (7): 1084-1093. https://doi.org/10.1038/ajg.2017.101.